Health Without Hospitals
The Healing Power of Nature

First Edition
Volume One

Christie C. Yerby, NMD
www.DrYerby.com

Disclaimer
The information compiled in this book is based upon the research and the personal and
professional experiences of the author. The information contained in this book is for
educational purposes only and is not recommended as a means of diagnosing or treating any
illness. Unless you knowingly undertake a self-care program*, matters concerning physical
and mental health should be supervised by a health practitioner knowledgeable in treating
that particular condition. The author does not prescribe any remedies or assume any
responsibility for those who choose to treat themselves.

Self-care programs using U. S. medical-grade products and formulas, plus access to detailed
product information, can be authorized by the reader by using the Dr. Yerby-approved
resources found at www.DSSorders.com/OHR. 1-877-846-7122
Account registration code CY411.

These are formulas without toxic additives, fillers, dyes, or sugars.

Management at DSS has agreed to follow the manufacturer's storage and handling
requirements until products are shipped to the patient / customer. This may include
temperature-control or safe supply turnover time (expiration dates).

ISBN-13: 978-1502565891
ISBN-10: 1502565897

ON THE COVER: Echinacea (*Echinacea purpurea*) – also known as Purple Coneflower

Numerous clinical studies have confirmed this plant's leaves and roots are useful in strengthening the
body's immune system as well as for prevention and natural treatment of colds and flu.

DEDICATION

I dedicate this first edition of *Health Without Hospitals* to my mother, June Yerby, who has been my best friend and support system through thick and thin, through health and high waters, and who is an example herself of preventive care and optimal 'health without hospitals'.

ACKNOWLEDGEMENTS AND THANKS

Thanks to Andrew Weil, MD, my first mentor in the field of natural medicine, who encouraged me in 1994 to proceed further into the world of 'health-caring'.

And to Christianne Northrup, MD, Dean Ornish, MD, and Julian Whitaker, MD - all of whose words helped to introduced me to and inspired me to know that there was an alternate way of making health care choices, other than surgery. They were the torch-carriers for *Health Without Hospitals.*'

Thanks to Michael Cronin, NMD, who created the first spring semester class at Southwest College of Naturopathic Medicine and Health Sciences in Tempe, Arizona, just in time for me to begin classes there in 1996.

Thanks, also to Robert Patterson, MD, who recruited me immediately after my graduation from naturopathic medical school, inviting me in 2001 to North Carolina to join his integrative medicine practice.

My thanks to the editors at the *Sanford Herald* newspaper in North Carolina for recognizing the need for and creating the 'Health and Science' page so that "The Healing Power of Nature" could be read each Sunday.

And my thanks especially to Terence Shepherd, my faithful friend and *'Wind Beneath my Wings'*, for always being there for me . . . since day one.

TABLE OF CONTENTS

ABOUT THE AUTHOR

Written in 2015

Dr. Yerby is a naturopathic physician, licensed in Arizona, the U.S. state considered to be the gold standard of licensing for naturopathic physicians due to the requirement to pass an additional full day of medical board tests necessary for the Arizona naturopathic medical license .

She is trained as a family medicine general practitioner and is board-tested in both the conventional medicines such as internal medicine, pathology, and pharmacology as well as the natural health sciences of clinical nutrition, botanical medicine, acupuncture, and others.

This degree is considered a double-track medical training, given that it includes a curriculum in both the conventional medical studies (such as required for MDs) and during the same four-years, the additional training and clinical hours in the natural health sciences.

She is a professional member of the American Association of Restorative Medicine, the American Association of Naturopathic Physicians, and the American Botanical Council.

Dr. Yerby is also certified in the NEI SuperSystem (Neurology-Endocrinology-Immune) established by NeuroScience Inc.

Her first mentor and advisor was Andrew Weil, MD, the 'Father of Integrative Medicine. She developed a relationship with him while studying the botanical medicines in the jungles of Tulum, Mexico, during an integrative medicine workshop he hosted. From there, after witnessing first hand from Dr. Weil the power of plant-based therapies, her interest in 'the healing power of nature' blossomed.

She continued and expanded her experiences and training on the healing potentials of natural medicines by closely observing other cultural non-drug systems of care with the medical doctors in the Bahamas, Jamaica, Hawaii, and Cuba. She visited Cuba three times as a medical student to observe within the hospitals and clinics their medical system, free of Western medicine's pharmaceuticals.

She has devoted her adult life to understanding the biochemical language of the natural sciences, making both personal and financial sacrifices, in order to bring the benefits of health without hospitals to an information-hungry public.

It is from these valued relationships and years of classroom studies and clinical practice that she can say with clarity and confidence that with the *healing power of nature* - we **can** receive . . . *health without hospitals.*

* * *

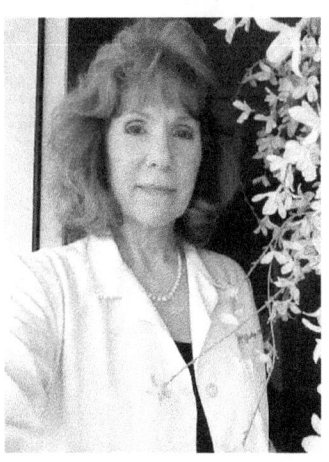

Christie C. Yerby, NMD
Naturopathic Medical Doctor, Author

PREFACE

Several years ago as a young woman, my gynecologist announced that I would have to have a full hysterectomy to alleviate some minor, yet aggravating symptoms. Surgery, I thought? I began researching my options. Much to my amazement, I discovered that there was, literally, a whole world of non-surgical options available to me.

My interest took me from one book to another and I have not stopped reading and researching since.

This change in my behavior won me the name of "Curious George" from my mother, as I became quite curious as to why more people did not realize that they had options and alternatives, empowering them to participate in making the right choices for their best healthcare. I became familiar with the name of board-certified gynecologist, Dr. Christianne Northrup, MD, whose information on natural solutions to women's health alerted me to the fact that word is not getting out fast enough regarding our choices. I vowed then to participate with others in raising awareness to help people make the informed decisions that are right for them.

Within the next few years, I met Dr. Johnathan Wright, MD, during an anti-aging conference, and studied briefly with Dr. Andrew Weil, MD, both of whom gave me further encouragement to pursue the path of what was then being called then "alternative medicine."

At age 46, through Divine direction and a wish and a prayer, I entered a pre-med program, then sold my lovely house in Kansas City (actually, Overland Park) and moved across the country by myself to an accredited naturopathic medical school. I sacrificed valuable time with family and friends to spend four years in Arizona obtaining the double-track medical education, costing me over $100,000, called naturopathic medicine.

Then, again by the Grace of God, I was 'brought' to North Carolina by special invitation to teach others what was happening in the world of science beyond that of conventional allopathic medicine – to share the same inspirational help that saved me from surgery and hospitals.

I have put to beneficial use my undergraduate degree in journalism by writing articles such as these to help reach those who may be looking for this help, but do not know where to find it.

So, here within these pages to follow, is a collection of some of those previously published articles from the "Healing Power of Nature" column – written by me as that new arrival to North Carolina - for the sole purpose of illuminating a new path, planting a seed, or changing a life.

By the way, I never did have the hysterectomy.

* * *

INTRODUCTION

OPEN LETTER TO READERS OF MY COLUMN…

As a columnist for the *Sanford Herald*'s 'Science and Health' page, you have "heard" me describe the choices that we have now in health care, the resources we have to help us access more information, and find support. Medicine today is changing fast, whether or not we can see it from our local vantage point. And despite who may agree or disagree with me, I have been chosen to carry the news of its arrival, whether by fate or by choice, or by God.

It is only by carrying the torch, passing it from one to another, that we will find and illuminate the main source of truth, gathering strength from numbers. It is through faith and desire that we seek the truth to begin with; it is with commitment and integrity that we want to stand up for it and represent it.

So, it is with medicine and healthcare these days. Once clear and decisive, the doctor's word was the final word; today this concept is not so defined. Who has the final word now? The insurance company? The pharmacist? The nurse? Or the doctor? The answer is unclear. One fact is for sure, though, when we lose the answers we lose our way. We find ourselves in the dark, we have no guides, and our health suffers.

What has happened to our *own* vote? True - safe dosage decisions and treatments plans are best left up to the medically-trained. Granted, those who have sacrificed so much to tend to our health are due our respect. Let us not forget, though, that it is a two way street, and we should not be hesitant to expect the same respect in return from them.

These are days when we should come to expect a partnership with our healthcare leaders. We are empowered and entitled to participate in the decisions and the plan of our care. That does not mean we talk back to our docs like derelicts and run rampant through the hall wearing nothing but our cotton gowns. It is to say, however, we should be alert and interested, listen closely, and get involved. We are in the end responsible for our own health - no one else.

We have many choices today. Conventional medicine takes us down the pharmaceutical and surgical paths as the answers to our illness. But success stories are springing up all over the country from those therapies not so conventional.

It is these stories that I want to share with you in future columns.

Having been a participant, myself, in healthcare in many parts of the world, and having been trained in a fully-credentialed school of naturopathic medicine, I hope to bring a new perspective to North Carolina by being a torchbearer for that greater source of illumination. It will not be of interested to everyone, only a source of light for those trying to find their way out of the darkness of ill health.

* * *

What would life be
if we had no courage to attempt anything?

VINCENT VAN GOGH
1853 – 1890
Dutch Painter

THE PHILOSOPHY

OVERVIEW: WHAT IS NATUROPATHIC MEDICINE?

There's a new style of medicine that is beginning to take the country by storm. It is grounded in traditional remedies of family heritage and customs, yet supported in truth and science by current clinical research. It is called "naturopathic medicine," and it seems to be here to stay.

Naturopathic medicine is often *incorrectly* called 'homeopathic medicine'. Homeopathy is a very limited choice of treatment originating in Germany. Think of naturopathic medicine as the complete system of natural medicine, with homeopathy being only one of many 'tools of treatment' available from which to choose by naturopathic doctors (as described later in this article).

Naturopathic medicine is the ultimate and complete 'healing power of nature' system of care, utilizing treatment resources provided by nature.

Naturopathic physicians stay abreast of current research constantly taking place in the ever-changing field of today's medicine, while always comparing it to the tried-and –true therapies we have learned from our forefathers.

One does not have to look too far to read that for years, now, medicine throughout the country has been leaning towards the return of "natural therapies". So, with one foot firmly embedded in the roots of the past, and the other balanced in the medical science of the future, naturopathic medicine was born.

One should also know the term, 'allopathic doctor' which refers to the conventional medical doctors (MD) most commonly found in medicine today. 'Allopathic' refers to doctors who treat symptoms only, and are not trained in the discovery of the causes or the preventions of chronic illnesses, such as with 'naturopathic' physicians.

Trained in four-year naturopathic medical schools, requiring a 2-year pre-med, curriculum, plus a 4-year undergraduate degree previous to that, naturopathic doctors must meet intense academic requirements to prepare them to accurately diagnose and treat patients.

They undergo the same thorough medical science education requirements as that of other medical doctors (MDs). Conventionally-trained MDs, however, do not receive within their training curriculum the natural health sciences courses (that naturopathic medicine does) such as medical nutrition, botanical (plant) medicine, homeopathy, physical medicine, counseling, oriental medicine (including acupuncture), hydrotherapy, detoxification, and more. Unfortunately, this leaves out a lot of 'health' from conventional healthcare.

Naturopathic physicians are trained as primary care general practitioners in preventing and treating chronic and degenerative diseases such as hypertension, chronic pain and fatigue, viral infections, high cholesterol, arthritis, heart disease, and cancer.

On top of their course training, they are required to do 1,200 hours of clinical internship working directly with patients in a clinical setting, as well as 40 hours of community service, and present findings of the research project study they personally designed and completed, before they are considered diploma-ready.

Emphasis is on "prevention" with the belief that given the opportunity, the encouragement, and supportive conditions, the body will rebalance and heal itself. They seek to restore the body to its overall optimal health and to prevent further illness through eliminating the underlying cause of the symptoms. Usually this is not the "quick fix" we have become accustomed to with current conventional medicine, but instead it is a gradual reshaping of life-style, and the adjusting of imbalances in the body, which over time, have created conditions in the body that often lead to illness.

NDs (or also knowns as NMDs) view disease symptoms as opportunities and indicators, clues to conditions that cry out for a holistic approach to treatment. This "whole person" patient approach assures a personalized plan, specific to the individual person, uniting both mind and body in its process of healing.

The use of diverse, non-intrusive, and essentially harmless methods, emphasizing the components of nature including those of sunlight, pure water and air, and nutritional products from the earth and sea, is the treatment philosophy of naturopathic doctors. They acknowledge the importance of emergency medicine to address the acute or life-threatening conditions and welcome the integrative collaboration and teamwork with conventional MDs, DOs, and DCs, each medical system complementing the other, in the goal to move a person into a state of long-term optimal health.

Empowering the patient to be responsible for his or her own health and well-being, naturopathic physicians are also teachers, encouraging a close partnership between doctor and patient to facilitate a safe and successful health program.

Many feel that naturopathic medicine is a long-overdue adjunct to today's medical system. There seems to be a breeze blowing across the hearts and minds of people full of the yearning to reconnect to the power and magic we once shared with the plants, the earth, and each other, to experience again the peace we get from "stopping to smell the roses." There is the want, and need, and yet there is the fear to change.

So, who will lead this pilgrimage back to a more naturally healthy life, the journey whose first step is the most important one? Who will reintroduce us to our "roots"? It will be those new docs on the horizon they call naturopathic doctors - those who seek energy from the warmth of the sun, who crave the purity of air and water, those who speak freely of the healing power of nature.

It is a journey open to all who choose it, a path accessible to everyone, just by taking that first step.

* * *

Simple Steps for a Long and Healthy Life

I am not a fan of TV commercials, especially when they boast the so-called health benefits of synthetic drugs and cheap, over-the-counter supplements that promise you the kitchen sink, including everything from A to Z.

But this one did catch my attention. It is of a woman saying, "If the woman of tomorrow could talk to the woman of today, she would say, 'Take care of yourself *now*.'

Never in the history of the world of advertising, has there been such valid advice, a message important to both men and women. Take the time right now to stop and think what you should be doing to assure that your health in ten, twenty, or thirty years will be the best it can be from your efforts today.

Preparing for physical health for the golden years is no different than preparing for financial health in later life. We often forget the former, yet understand the importance of the latter. Why is that?

Since most people do not often receive advise on how to achieve this optimal longevity from just their conventional, fast-paced, seven-minute-a-visit medical doctor, it is important to find either a naturopathic physician, plus an MD, or DC that understands the philosophy of integrative medicine, and include them in your network of health resources, in order to get "the rest of the story." Often the cost of this balance of information comes directly out of your pocket, but paying for your personal health maintenance is well worth it. Put your money into something that will give you life. After all, what could be more important?

Whether man or woman, whether age 40, 50, 60, or 70, or older it is time to make the changes you know you need to make, to assure that the "older you" is the best it can be. It is easier to prevent a problem than it is to fix it. Start now.

Here are some essentials to consider:

Number one, of course, is stop smoking. This is the best health gift you can give to yourself. If you do nothing else for yourself and your family, do this. This includes removing yourself from the exposure to secondhand smoke, and eliminating the habit of tobacco chewing.

22

Stop eating sugar and artificial sweeteners. Many ill-health conditions are related to sugar and the toxicities of aspartame, saccharin, and sucralose (Splenda®). Use the plant-based, stevia, instead.

Reduce your red meat intake, especially if it is cooked over an open flame (cancer-causing), or contains a lot of fat. Dietary fat is absorbed through your lymphatic system in the digestive process; the lymphatic system empties into your heart and coronary artery system.

Center your diet on a rainbow of whole natural foods including the reds, yellows, greens, oranges, and blues that are strong in vitamins and minerals, while avoiding white foods that are starchy, processed, and lack nutritional value.

Don't drink chlorinated tap water. Despite the safety claims, there have still been reports of health violations. Pesticides can leach into water supplies, as can bacteria, and harmful elements both from the water itself and the pipe system can be carried from the original water source to your glass. Drink distilled or filtered water instead. Remember to eat foods rich in organic minerals in order to replace those eliminated from distillation or filtration, such as calcium and magnesium.

Slow down, breathe, and smile. Match your pace with the speed-of-nature, not the artificial one of modern technology. We were born into God's world of plants, clouds, and gentle breezes, and are an integral part of that environment. We have come to know, instead, and have attached ourselves to 80-miles-an-hour on the highway, fast foods, bright lights, and loud, crowded checkout counters. Redirect your mind and your perspective to include the healing powers of nature. Your heart will thank you.

Be thankful and forgive. As total long-term health includes body, mind, and spirit let us not forget the benefits derived from counting our blessings. Be thankful for what you have today, not worrying about losses of yesterday, or what may or may not bear fruit tomorrow.

Take care of today and tomorrow will take care of itself. In addition, forgive those who you think may have crossed you; chances are they have long ago forgotten their transgression, leaving you still hurting from your own angry label of the mishap. Many people claim that their pent up anger, sadness, and anxiety has led to their cancer. Leave ill thoughts in the past where they belong and move on to healthier days. The only reality is today's reality.

Avoid toxic elements. This includes breathing bad air, taking excessive synthetic drugs, avoiding negative or deceptive people, and eliminating overexposure to sun and other radiation, excessive alcohol, and processed tobacco. Our livers, lungs, and kidneys can only handle only so much before they quit clearing the poisons.

And despite recent talk that blood tests / lab work is a waste of time and money, I strongly disagree. Getting regular blood work, obtaining your own copy of the report, and knowing the basics of how to read it is invaluable for monitoring a possible developing health concern. Ask your doctor to assist you in this, your desire to learn more about your health.

Surprisingly, staying strong into later life is not achieved with a drawer full of prescribed drugs or sacks of discount store supplements, but consists of having faith in the simple acts of living in the natural world into which we were born.

No matter of what age you are, or in what stage of health you may be, begin now to build towards health in future years, begin now to reverse the damage, begin now to invest in your health.

This is the You-of-Tomorrow speaking to the You-of-Today saying, "Take care of yourself . . . *now*."

* * *

INCURABLE PEOPLE: JUST MY OPINION

Recently, I was asked if naturopathic doctors "cure" diabetes. I replied that in our training of naturopathic medicine, we are taught that there are no incurable diseases, only incurable people.

It is just my opinion, but by becoming aware of the many healthcare options now available, of which there are many (other than the use of conventional pharmaceutical drugs), you may save your life or the one of a loved one.

The phrase, "think globally, act locally," applies not only to environmental awareness, but also to healthcare, as many effective treatment choices originated in India, China, Japan, Europe, and from the Native American Indians, not K-Mart or Wal-Mart. Ignoring the power of centuries-old global medicines, by only "thinking locally," may limit your healthcare options, restricting you to what is available at a local drugstore or discount store.

Some of the worldwide universal therapies include botanical (herbal) medicine, which saved the lives of many prior to the establishment of the pharmaceutical industry, and is still doing so; hydrotherapy, using water and its movement and heat variations to improve immune system function; and medical nutrition, applying the basic tenants of biochemistry to improve human deficiencies.

It is the "incurable" conditions, which are often benefited most by these "alternative" resources. Those who deny the existence or benefits of these natural methods, which reach beyond drug therapy, may be the incurable people, as their mindset may not permit their health to take that life-saving turnaround it perhaps could.

To doubt the powerful effects of plant nutrients on the human body is to lack knowledge of biochemistry, nothing more. To dispute the existence of metabolic reactions that the addition of organic nutrients has on the human body (either from food or supplement form) is again, falling short of having basic information on the nutritional sciences.

Those that do not know what the Krebs Cycle of human metabolism is, will naturally not understand what role the addition of quality supplements, or carefully chosen foods, may play in medicine. It is from this vast puzzle of biochemistry terms, symbols, and lengthy words that many answers to incurable diseases will be found. But only a trained translator educated in human biochemistry can determine what is missing from that picture, in order to suggest a fitting solution.

From within this wired-wizardry of the human machinery called biochemistry, a professional trained in 'functional medicine' can often identity a missing nutrient, enzyme, or hormone - the very one that could be the important building block of a key ingredient needed to produce "the cure" of a so-called incurable disease. By understanding the biochemical pathways to human healing through the study of this 'basic' medical science, the answers to resolving the most difficult of ailments are often found.

Very few conventionally trained medical doctors receive the extensive training on the biochemistry of human metabolism that would qualify them to unlock the biochemical codes, which ultimately relates directly to the alterations needed to correct, not just medicate, health deficiencies. Most of them are not even interested in knowing.

However, those doctors who *are* interested in getting to the "source of the problem," undergo a lengthy training, racking up hundreds of hours of classroom and clinical training on this specialty. These are the medically trained naturopathic doctors of today, licensed from only four accredited naturopathic medical schools in the U.S. and two in Canada It is from this double-track medical science curriculum that their natural medicine practices are based.

Without faith, little can be achieved. Understandably, information on current world research is not always easily accessible locally. But without acknowledgment that the pool of information from which you are basing your opinion may be less than complete, expansion, growth, and perhaps healing, may be impossible.

'Just my opinion, but if you are fortunate to know that there are tremendous resources available for even the most difficult-to-cure conditions, you are already plugged in to the resources and rewards of natural global medicines.

If instead, you are still forming your opinions and making your health decisions by what you are reading on the labels at a discount store, perhaps a little more interest would help save your life - or that of someone you love.

* * *

Ignore your health, and it will go away.

LAYING CLAIM TO OPTIMAL HEALTH

"There's nothing I can do about it."

How does it feel to hear those words from your doctor? The finality of these words destroys all options for a creative or possible alternative. It is an easy answer for him, a quick answer and one that shuffles the situation under the rug making less room for a hopeful 'tomorrow'. It is a statement we do not want to hear from our doctor, and yet it is one we freely use ourselves... *for* ourselves.

The beliefs about our genetic make-up may lead us to take a complacent attitude toward our own heath, unfortunately, reducing the tomorrows for which we had hoped.

It is easy to roll over and say, "Yes, I have heart disease; it is in my family. Pass the French fries." Or, "I gain weight no matter how little candy I eat; it is in my genes." Astonishing as it may seem, however, the fat that is now in the heart, and the sugar that has settled around the waist was not due to any predisposition of heredity, but instead to a lack to self-responsibility towards our own optimal health.

It has not been long ago that popular thought maintained that 'you are what your genes say you are', like it or not. But more recently, both NDs (naturopathic doctors) and MDs are agreeing that despite our genetic selection, we ultimately are our own healthcare decision-makers.

Ray McKnight, MD, Truman Medical Center in Key West, Florida, describes our choices, "*We* are the masters of our own health and well-being," he says. He subscribes to the doctrine that genetic predisposition is merely an "option" and that these traits do not necessarily manifest.

"The wholeness of our own unique selves has the greatest potential to affect our health – gene or no gene," McKnight says. "There is a part of us that exists beyond our body," he states.

Others agree. Lendon H. Smith, MD, author of *Feed Your Body Right*, is convinced that, "Though fate may have handed you some negative genetic traits, many of them may be offset." In his book, Dr. Smith says, "While genes determine your susceptibility to certain diseases, it is clear that such diseases need not become manifest unless your lifestyle – including several factors, chiefly diet – allow them to surface."

There appears to be plenty of scientific literature to support these ideas. From the *Archives of Internal Medicine* (1998; 158: 698-704), researchers at the University of Helsinki, Finland, say ulcers may be caused more by environmental factors than genetics. In this issue, Dr. Ismo Raiha reported that smoking and stress in men and analgesics in women attributed to an increase risk of ulcers. Environmental (lifestyle) factors accounted for 61 percent of ulcer development while genetics accounted for the other 39 percent, the study reports.

A recent report from the *New England Journal of Medicine* supports the idea that the role of the environment may be more powerful than the role of genes in influencing whether one develops cancer. The study tracked cancer patterns in 400,000 identical twins in Scandinavia. The question was: If one twin developed cancer, what were the chances that the other twin with the same genetic material would also develop the same cancer. For most common types of cancer, including lung, breast, and colorectal, the chance that the identical twin would develop the same cancer as that of the afflicted one, was just 15%.

Those who applaud the attempts of drug therapy to correct the *cause* of illness should remember that, by definition, the role of naturopathic medicine *is* to address the cause of disease. But marketing of genetic code altering drugs by pharmaceutical companies (who will be paying for this data) is, however, apparently on the horizon via the Human Genome Project.

We have digressed and forgotten much of the writings from the traditional medicines of the early 1900s, when there were no "gene-altering" pharmaceuticals upon which to fall. From *Biochemistry of Schuessler*, 1920, Dr. Wilhelm Heinrich Schuessler wrote from Chapter I: Vis Medicatrix Naturae (The Healing Power of Nature), "The human machine is self-building, self-cleansing, self-repairing and self-destroying."

Each of us must decide for ourselves which philosophy to endorse when making decisions for our own health: support and allow for the healing power of nature, or utilize the results of recent medical science in the form of synthetic drug therapy to effect a change….a tough choice for many.

But despite which side of the fence one is on regarding the role genetics is playing in their health, and how to manage its effects, it is safe to say that if we do not fall prey to an "out-of-my-hands" attitude, we may all be able to lay claim to optimal health.

* * *

HEART HEALTH

KNOW YOUR NUMBERS: CHOLESTEROL AWARENESS

Cholesterol has gotten a bad reputation, perhaps unjustly.

Certainly, with heart disease reported as being the number one health problem in this country we need to use caution and watch our cholesterol. The cholesterol number, however, is not the only number to watch.

Lipitor®, the most often prescribed drug for lowering cholesterol, can often bring a cholesterol number down quickly returning it to its so-called 'safe range', protecting the arteries from potential damage from fatty plaque buildup, and thus from heart attacks and stroke. It is interesting, however, that in the process of protecting the heart from damage with this and other "statin" drugs, the very nutrient needed for heart and muscle health and energy production is depleted. This is common knowledge for those health care professionals who are aware of nutrient depletions caused by drug therapy.

Monitoring cholesterol is important, especially for those living a sedentary lifestyle and eating junk foods. But even more important is monitoring other blood lipids - the triglycerides, the LDLs, and the HDLs. Knowing these numbers will provide a much better picture of heart health than cholesterol alone.

There are other valuable blood tests that can help define heart health, too, but these are lesser known and much less often ordered by the doctor. They are hs-CRP (high sensitivity C-reactive protein), homocysteine, and LDL particle size. Asking your doctor about these may support his interest in ordering them, and knowing the results, as well.

I worked with a man with normal cholesterol levels who had a family history of heart disease. He thought he was safe from what he perceived would be his genetic fate, heart disease. When completing a blood test evaluation with a "full lipid panel," and the other heart health blood tests, he was surprised to find that his cardiac risk was dangerously high due to other parameters that had never been tested, much less monitored. Knowing these numbers and taking steps to correct them may have saved his life.

So, know your numbers, but know *all* your numbers. Have your doctor explain the importance of each lipid (cholesterol) value until you understand their importance to your health.

Those who decline the pharmaceutical answers to blood lipid controls have choices available to them. The treatment will vary depending on the elevated lab value needing to be lowered the most. These are common pharmaceutical grade nutrients that, in therapeutic dosages, have been clinically studied to result in a reduction of excessive animal fat foods in the blood.

Some doctors feel that high LDLs and triglycerides are more dangerous than high cholesterol. I agree with them given the fact that cholesterol may normally be a little high in some people, which may call for little to no pharmaceutical intervention.

With all other blood lipids well within the normal range, a high cholesterol report might best be addressed by changing to a diet low in animal fat coupled with the appropriate therapeutic nutrients.

Rarely mentioned is the importance of cholesterol to our good health and well-being. Most people do not know that cholesterol is a steroid hormone produced in the liver ('...sterol'). It is from cholesterol that other hormones are produced including estrogen, testosterone, and vitamin D. Postmenopausal women whose bodies are desperately trying to produce estrogen are very likely to have high cholesterol. It is quite possibly not due to heart disease developing; the liver is just trying to produce more estrogen in an estrogen-depleted woman.

Unfortunately, some doctors insist on lowering a slightly elevated cholesterol in women (up to 235). This can create even more estrogen-deficient symptoms by causing a further depletion in estrogen levels. Rarely do doctors take into consideration a women's age or hormone-producing ability before he writes out that prescription for a statin drug. They do what I call 'lab reference medicine'. One size, one age, fits all. Certainly check the other tests if you are worried about heart disease, however.

(In addition, men whose cholesterol levels have been medically lowered to 'safe levels' may unnecessarily experience symptoms related to low testosterone.)

A cholesterol number that is naturally very low (under 140) could indicate an underactive liver, such as a fatty-liver, and possibly restrict its ability to make these important hormones.

Bottom line: when it comes to cholesterol and other blood lipids, know *all* your numbers, or before you know it, *your* number may be up!

* * *

Watch for Dr. Yerby's book:
"Keeping Tabs on Your Labs"
. . . a simple guide to translating the results of your blood work.

When Diet and Exercise are Not Enough

There was an interesting full-page ad in the *New York Times* recently.

The ad contained warnings, precautions, and side effect advisories for a swallowed item if it did not have careful medical observation and monitoring, lab work, and close follow-up. This was not an ad for rat poisoning; it was an ad for the cholesterol-lowering medicine, Zocor®.

The ad on this report was addressed to the attention of the users of the cholesterol-lowering drug, Baycol®. If you did not catch the national news at that time, you need to know that this statin drug was removed from the market after 31 deaths in this country were reported that were linked to an unusual side effect from taking the drug.

What Merck does not say in their ad, however, is that Zocor®, as well as Mevacor®, Prevachol®, Lescol®, and Lipitor® are all in the same class of "statin" drugs as Baycol®. The same adverse effects apply to all of them, according to physician's *Drugs Facts and Comparisons* reference guide, which advises patients to report promptly any "muscle pain, tenderness or weakness, particularly with malaise (fatigue) or fever," while taking any of these drugs.

According to the USA Today, Bayer's Baycol® was linked to significantly more fatal cases of rhabdomyolysis (breakdown of muscle tissue resulting in kidney damage) than the other statin drugs and that this side effect was most likely to occur when Baycol® was given in high doses, or when it was given with another cholesterol-lowering drug, Lopid® (gemfibrozil). The article goes on to say that despite the agreement between Bayer and the FDA to change the drug's labels advising doctors not to prescribe the drugs together, many still did.

Granted, statin drugs may be a life-saving participant when arteries are 90% blocked, as was the case for the model featured in the ad text. But when lipids are slightly to moderately high and family history is not saturated with heart disease, perhaps there are other choices.

Doctors trained in the alternative medicine sciences know that there are now clinically researched nutrients from which to select. These not only accomplish cholesterol-lowering results, they may also support other body systems favorably.

An herb from India, Guggul (*Commiphora mukul)*, has shown no significant adverse effects reported in clinical trials, according to the editors of the *Pharmacist's Letter in their Natural*

Medicine Comprehensive Database Book. This botanical medicine has also been used for weight loss, as it is said to have thyroid-stimulating properties.

A common B vitamin, pantethine (vitamin B5), has been shown through studies to be one of the most effective natural agents at therapeutic doses for lowering triglycerides without adverse side effects. In fact, other conditions that may be helped at the same time with pantethine is chronic fatigue, allergies, wound healing, rheumatoid or osteoarthritis, depression, Lupus, and athletic performance.

A favorite choice for many doctors already is the use of niacin (vitamin B3) for lowering cholesterol. As with other natural agents, the proper form of the vitamin is important. The non-flushing form is most popular for lowering lipids. Due to niacin's effect on the circulation system, other benefits from taking this vitamin may be improved memory, help with acne, better digestion, protection from toxins and pollutants, and help in lowering blood pressure.

Although natural in origin, these supplements are not to be taken without direction from a doctor trained in the natural sciences, as too much of a good thing is still not a good thing. Proper dosing specific to each individual's past and present medical history is essential. Interactions with other drugs and supplements can still occur, even with products marked "natural," although usually not life-threatening as we've recently seen between synthetic drugs.

For those wanting to follow the instructions described within the Zocor® ad, advising patients to use this drug "as an addition to diet," when diet and exercise are not enough, they post a great food list and exercise program on their website. Lipitor® has similar help on theirs.

As these statin drugs are effective for other cardiac conditions, consult a doctor about your situation before making any decisions on your own. As the ad says, ask your doctor what is right for you. It does not hurt, however, to couple that with a little research on your own.

* * *

THE CARBS VS. FATS DEBATE

Would you pour that white, thick, left-over-from-cooking fat down your kitchen sink? No, it would stop up the pipes. Then, why would we want to pour the same thing into our arteries? These are 'solid' fats, usually from animal meat sources, and are a contributing factor to heart disease.

Udo Erasmus (udoerasmus.com), the internationally recognized authority on the subject of fats and oils, says of saturated fats: "An *excess* of saturated fatty acids can cause health problems for our hearts and arteries." They are "sticky, sluggish molecules", he says, that can be deposited within cells, organs, and arteries, encouraging platelets to stick together, plaguing especially those people whose diets are high in animal foods like beef, pork, dairy products (cheese and whole milk).

Diets high in refined sugars can also create cardiovascular problems, in part because our body converts excess sugar into saturated fats, storing it if it is not used, often-increasing triglycerides and cholesterol levels. Triglycerides from sugars are especially a health problem when they have been "oxidized" due to lack of antioxidant minerals and vitamins in a diet.

You say you don't eat much sugar? How about the juice and bagels or toast for breakfast, then a sandwich for lunch? Potato, corn, or rice for dinner? All are carbohydrates. Once digestion begins, they become a sugar form in the body, ready to be used for energy for those after-meals walks we all do, or to be stored as fat if we go straight to the TV set, the computer, or on to bed.

Let us not get the 'fats that kill' mixed up with the 'fats that heal', though. Let's see, there are the EFAs, the MCTs, and the GLAs. Then there are the LAs, the LNAs, and the EPAs. When does it ever end? Just give me my hamburger and hush up, already! We all have heard confusing stories about how fats, oils, cholesterol, and nutrients affect our health. One says this, the other says that; we are screaming for a simple and clear understanding, and we're not going to take it any longer!

Most medical and naturopathic doctors agree that it is not necessarily the eating of the fats, but the altering of the fats once in the body, that does the most damage. That is why diets high in fats need support from a selection of special nutrients, specific for prevention of the changing of these fats into fats that kill. These are the antioxidants.

These nutrient co-factors include support from elements that help "metabolize", or keep moving, the fat from the cells and muscle to a place it can be used as energy. Without enough of these nutritional supportive measures, during high fat consumption, fat may travel to the arteries of the heart where it could stay.

How can fats that kill get stuck in the arteries around the heart? Unlike proteins and carbohydrates from the food we eat that go to the liver first from the intestines through capillaries, fats go to *the heart first*, by getting absorbed by the lymph system from the digesting intestines. Pretty boring anatomical information, and well-hidden in medical textbooks, it is the best-kept secret that could save someone from developing heart disease.

So, what are the right foods to avoid for the healthiest heart, carbs or fats? The debate goes on. It is not a rubber-stamp answer, but a lengthy study of medical nutrition. The simple basics, though, if you are not very active you are to avoid the sugary foods, starchy carbs/vegetables, the very sweet fruits, and the animal fats that have the thick, white marbling.

Remember that high fat diets require fat-metabolizing nutritional help for safety from igniting of damaging reactions (free radicals) to cells, arteries, and organs, and that excess intake of any of these foods will store as triglycerides and cholesterol if not used for energy. That's pretty much it, in a fat cell.

Though complex and advanced, this topic is well worth your own personal study and essential if you have heart disease in your family.

And one last simple reminder: Do not pour into your own pipes, what you would not dispose of in your own kitchen.

* * *

TOXICITY

NUTRITIONAL SUPPLEMENTS TO DIE FOR

It is amazing the amount of toxins that are in some nutritional supplements these days. Perhaps it was by the example of the food industry that originally sanctioned it as being OK, that other industries feel that they can follow. Now, even some of our nutritional supplements, the sacred resource we have trusted as being "good for us", is causing concern.

What we eat as food, swallow as supplement and drug pill coatings or medicinal syrups, or rub on ourselves as cosmetics often contain toxic coal-tar based dyes. According to several resources on the subject four of these dyes, Red 3, Yellow 5, Yellow 6, and Blue 2, have been shown to cause cancer, as have other dyes, which are not used in food, but are used in drugs or cosmetics.

Fortunately, the history of food dyes in the U.S. is one of "decreasing" rather than "increasing." Of the 24 food dyes previously allowed in the American food supply, 17 are now banned, de-listed, or no longer produced. We are, however, still waiting for the other seven to be removed from consumer products by the FDA. Until then, we continue to consume them.

Toxicity of three dyes (Red 3, Yellow 5, and Yellow 6) is the subject of a Public Citizen Health Research Group petition to the FDA, calling for a ban. The group has also reviewed the safety studies on the other four dyes (Green 3, Red 40, Blue 1, and Blue 2), because of previous toxic findings.

FD&C Blue No. 2 was shown to produce malignant tumors at the site of injection when introduced under the skin of rats. The World Health Organization gives it a toxicology rating of B, meaning that data was not sufficient to make it acceptable for food use.

FD&C Yellow No. 6 is used in food, alcohol, supplements, cosmetics, and hair rinses. In 1986, the FDA passed a ruling that it had to be listed on the labels because of its ability to cause allergic reactions. Don't be fooled, though. Check your one-a-day "A to Z" vitamins and you will note that the dyes are listed only on the outer throw-away box, and not on the inside bottle label itself that you keep and show your doctor for his safety approval.

Tests conducted on FD&C Red No. 40 were all conducted by its manufacturer, (name withheld). Consequently, many American scientists feel that the safety of Red No. 40 is far from established. The National Cancer Institute reported that *p*-credine, a chemical used in preparation of Red No. 40, was carcinogenic in animals. In rats, a high dose caused adverse reproductive effects.

[FD&C stands for the FDA regulated categories most commonly using these dyes in their products or formulas - 'food, drugs, and cosmetics.']

Aspirin-sensitive patients have been reported to develop life-threatening asthmatic symptoms when ingesting Yellow No. 5. By law, it too is supposed to be on the label when added to a product. But, again, many products do not reflect these additives if the lists of ingredients are not labeled directly on the bottle. Watch for this.

Of particular interest, these toxic dyes are not only being read from the labels of junk foods, candies, and fertilizers, they are coming right off the outside boxes of a popular multivitamin for kids. Oh, and one more interesting thing, it adds on the back of the vitamin product box: *"Keep out of reach of children."*

* * *

The only medicine for suffering, crime,
and all other woes of mankind
is wisdom.

THOMAS HENRY HUXLEY

WHEN "SWEET" IS NOT SO SWEET

The sweet fact is this: sugar is killing us. Our strong desire to eat sweets has to stop if we are to live a long and healthy life.

Pure white processed sugar, whether being added to foods and drinks, or already in them is ruining our health and is a contributor to making our country one plagued with obesity, cancer, and fatigue. Sugar depletes our immune system, making us more vulnerable to illnesses. It gives us cavities, puts weight on us, feeds cancer cells, yeasts, and bacteria, and makes us tired. And even though it puts a smile on our faces, and satisfies a desire, it is actually a poison.

What is the alternative? The artificial sweeteners are worse. Aspartame, found in many foods, drinks, and nutritional supplements for kids, has been reported to cause seizures, headaches, and blackouts. Aspartame is available on the tabletops of most restaurants in the blue package. Common side effects linked to aspartame include dizziness, numbness of extremities, loss of equilibrium, disorientation, visual impairment, episodes of high blood pressure, and tunnel vision.

Next to it, in the pink package, you may find the cancer-causing sweetener that keeps you from being anything but "in the pink." Saccharin *should* display a warning disclaimer on its package exposing its cancer-causing qualities, even though it would be difficult to read on its small pink wrapper. Saccharin is a petroleum derivative that is a "co-carcinogen" (a promoter of cancer-causing agents in the body).

When high-sugar foods are eaten alone, blood sugar levels rise quickly, giving us a quick energy "up," then crashes down with a heavy fatigue response. Read food labels carefully for clues on sugar content. If the words dextrose, barley malt, sucrose, glucose, maltose, lactose, fructose, corn syrup, or white grape juice concentrate appears on the label, extra sugar has been added.

Before the 1970s, sugar beets and sugar cane were the largest source of sugar we consumed, but starting in the '70s, sugars produced from corn became more popular and less expensive to produce, giving many of us the same food allergy symptoms that corn often does.

In addition to food allergies, sugar may also be the contributing health factor in many other illnesses. Just some conditions that may be related to excess sugar consumption include: aggressive and irritable behavior, chronic infections and fatigue, arthritis, cancer, diabetes, vaginal inflammations, and heart disease.

Not only has virtually all the vitamin and mineral content been removed from white sugar, but even the smallest amount of sugar can inhibit the absorption of some vital nutrients that we do get, those needed for energy and good immune-system health, such as the B vitamins and zinc.

Here are some suggestions for helping you eliminate sugar from your life: Read the labels on everything, including nutritional supplements. (You will be surprised to see how much sugar is found there.) Stop adding sugar to your tea and coffee. Use stevia instead. (Truvia®) If you crave sweets, you may not be eating enough protein. With a properly balanced diet, your sugar cravings may diminish. Exercise. Exercising affects the appetite control center in the brain, making you fell less starved and less likely to want a "sugar fix."

The best choices to make these days are products made from the Chinese fruit, Lo Han Kuo, or stevia, a small plant grown in Paraguay. Lo Han Kuo is a natural sugar that has the least effect on insulin production than other natural sugar forms.

Stevia is made from a small shrub belonging to the Astor family of plants. Its leaves produce a very sweet taste, but have no caloric effect. It contains iron, calcium, zinc, vitamin C, vitamin A, and more. Stevia is still relatively unheard of in some parts of the country, in part due to the competitive "politics' within the sweetener industry.

If you have not been feeling or acting very "sweetly" lately, check your sugar consumption. We are what we eat, but we are not necessarily sweet from the sweets that we eat.

* * *

THE SWEET LIFE

Who would think that something so good, so sweet, so tempting, would dare try to harm us? Is it fair that our health should have to suffer when we are only trying to satisfy our cravings? Unfortunately, one of the sweetest things of life, sugar, does harm us.

While white sugar, fructose, honey, maple syrup, and corn syrup all qualify as "natural sweeteners", none of these are calorie-free nor can people who suffer from blood sugar disorders use them. They encourage weight gain, tooth decay, rise in blood sugar, and can also predispose certain individuals to yeast infections, and can aggravate arthritis.

Sugar can also contribute to indigestion, a rise in triglycerides as well as cholesterol, bowel disorders, hyperactivity, and possibly Attention Deficient Disorder (ADD), and ear infections in children. Sugar contributes to learning difficulties as well as aggressive behavior in children as well as in adults. Studies have shown that criminals put on a sugar-free diet became less violent. Sugar can lead to anxiety and depression.

Sugar leads to mineral deficiency, especially chromium, the most important mineral for the control of the blood sugar.

What about the other "natural sweeteners"? Fructose is somewhat better than sugar, but has been shown to deplete us of copper, an important mineral for the cardiovascular and immune system. Many people are sensitive to fructose, which can cause them to have stomach aches and loose bowels.

Honey and maple syrup are better than white sugar, but will also contribute to hyperglycemia (high blood sugar) and can cause intestinal yeast to grow. Additionally, some people are allergic to honey, and it can be dangerous for diabetics who have to avoid high blood sugar (glucose).

Brown sugar? Since raw sugar is susceptible to spoilage, refining produces a product more than 99.9% pure white sucrose with all vitamins and minerals removed. Due to the dangers of microbial contamination, it was also made unlawful to sell any sugar less refined. Thus, all apparently partly refined sugars such as brown sugars are actually made by adding molasses to refined white sugar.

One of the most disturbing and little-known facts about sugar is regarding its damaging effects it has on our immune system. Eating too much sugar can actually compromise our immune system by lowering the white blood cell count, making us more susceptible for disease. It contributes to the reduction in defense against bacterial infection. Neutrophils are the body's most abundant type of white blood cells, whose function is to destroy microorganisms in the body that cause disease, such as viruses and bacteria. Without adequate numbers of these, our body's defense against disease is lessened.

Sodas supply most of the sugar in our diets. Sugar added to cereals, teas, and coffee can also add up fast. Baked foods like cookies, breads, pies, and jellies add even more sugar to our intake. Even foods like catsup are loaded with sugar.

The amount of sugar we consume can have a profound effect on both our physical and mental well-being. Sugar is a powerful substance, which can have drug-like effects and is considered addictive by some nutritional experts (refer to *Sugar Blues* by William Duffy). In excess, sugar can be toxic and rob us of our vitamins.

Significant amounts of B vitamins are required to metabolize and detoxify sugar from our bodies. B vitamins are important nutrients the body needs to produce energy. Without sufficient amounts, we may tend to feel fatigued. And even though it appears we can get a quick rush of energy from sugar, we can be left feeling worse than before we consumed it, with our immune systems damaged and our nutrients depleted.

And the artificial sweeteners are even worse. These are among the most troubling of food additives on the market, even though they have been given the FDA stamp of approval. Apparently, worse than food additives, these chemicals can cause serious illnesses. Saccharin (Sweet 'N Low®) is a known carcinogen (causes cancer). In 1978 the National Academy of Sciences evaluated documentation from studies on saccharin and concluded that it promotes cancer-causing agents (a "co-carcinogen").

As word spread about saccharin, another artificial sweetener was developed - aspartame (Equal®), presently used in over 5,000 products. This is a combination of two amino acids (natural substances) and methanol (wood alcohol: *not* a natural substance.) Methanol is, in fact, poisonous even when consumed in relatively small amounts. The methanol in the aspartame converts to formaldehyde in the retina of the eye. Formaldehyde is grouped in the same class of drugs as cyanide and arsenic, deadly poisons.

Few long-term studies have been conducted on aspartame, but the FDA and the Centers for Disease Control indicate that continual consumption of aspartame in large amounts may affect our health. Three 12-ounce cans of diet cola contain as much as eight times the Environmental Protection Agency's recommended limit for methanol consumption.

The most common complaints from overuse of aspartame are dizziness, numbing of the hands and feet, inflammation of the pancreas and heart muscle, high blood pressure, visual problems, and seizures/behavioral problems. (The phenylalanine in aspartame breaks down the seizure threshold and depletes serotonin, which causes manic depression, panic attacks, rage, and violence.)

Aspartame appears to be especially dangerous to children and unborn babies. And for diabetics, aspartame is deadly. The aspartame keeps their blood sugar levels out of control causing many patients to go into a coma or even death. Their retinopathy is often created by aspartame.

Memory loss is due to the fact that aspartic acid and phenylalanine are neurotoxic without the other amino acids found in protein. When it passes the blood-brain barrier, aspartame deteriorates the neurons of the brain, causing brain damage of varying degrees. For this reason, aspartame is said to be escalating Alzheimer's disease.

Aspartame is found in diet foods and many other products, such as prepared foods and medicine. Use caution if the label reads "Sugar Free". Read your labels carefully and eliminate these items if they contain aspartame: instant teas, yogurt, frozen desserts, multi-vitamins, laxatives, cereals, instant breakfasts, cocoa mixes, juice beverages and sugar-free chewing gums to name a few.

Sucralose (Splenda®) is a combination of toxic chlorine and methanol chemicals. It was originally planned to be marketed as a *pesticide,* but when one of the researchers accidentally heard he was to 'taste it', instead of 'test it', they found it to be sweet and decided that more money could be made marketing it as a sweetener instead of as a pesticide. *("The Sweet Deception,"* by Mercola and Pearsall is a *must read.*) Cancers have been related to over-use.

While aspartame, saccharin, and sucralose continue to dominate the non-caloric sweetener scene, a remarkable herb called *stevia rebaudiana* remains less well known. (Ask for it at the store where you shop under the name Truvia®.) The leaves of the stevia plant contain glycosides that produce a sweet taste, but have no caloric value. Consequently, it will not cause weight gain, nor will it initiate a rise in blood sugar, nor promote bacterial growth.

Stevia is a small shrub that belongs to the Astor plant family and grows in the mountains of Paraguay. For centuries, this herbal sweetener has been used by native cultures to counteract the bitter taste of various plant-based medicines and beverages (their bush medicine). Stevia is not a food additive and not an artificial sweetener. Toxicology studies have been done in Japan, where it is used extensively, and determined to be safe. (Inquire at the store for products they carry.)

According to a report from the Hiroshima School of Dentistry, stevia actually suppresses the bacteria that cause dental decay, as opposed to feeding it. It has been used in South America as a tonic for physical and mental fatigue, to aid weight loss, regulate blood pressure, and improve digestion. The American FDA has also recognized it as safe, but is still not labeling it as a sweetener or food enhancer, even though it is many times sweeter than sugar. Perhaps politics plays a role in this.

For the sweetest *and* longest life, read your labels, avoid sugar intake, and don't consume the "artificials". Remember, all that glitters is not gold, and all that is sweet is not necessarily good.

* * *

THE CLEAR FACTS ON WATER

Water, water, everywhere, and still wondering what to drink…

No matter how well we take care of ourselves, no matter how good the quality of the supplements, or how much exercise we get, if we drink contaminated water, it all still goes down the toilet.

Water is beginning to be offered in such a vast variety that its section in the stores is beginning to rival that of soft drinks. Isn't water, just water? Why so many choices?

The cheapest and most available, of course, is hard (public) water. Even though city tap water is supposed to be frequently tested and does contain chorine, it may still occasionally contain bacteria, lead, and other disease-causing organisms. And, well water contains lots of minerals, but is also vulnerable to radon and pesticides from the soil. (Remember, whatever we consume as minerals in water, the kidney has to deal with, since the entire blood supply of our body passes through the kidneys and is filtered 15 times each hour.)

Problems with dehydration may not be the causative factor of all medical problems, but insufficient water intake and drinking impure water over a period of time, may just be the reason some of us feel just a little worse today than yesterday. By drinking distilled water rather than tap or well water we can often see a reversal of some health difficulties. The result can be joints that are less stiff, arteries more elastic, kidney and gallstones start to dissolve, and the stomach pains start to diminish.

"Noninfectious, recurring, or chronic pains should be viewed as indicators of body thirst," says F. Batmanghelidj, M.D., author of *Your Body's Many Cries for Water.*

It is easy to become dehydrated, especially in the middle of the summer. A common misconception that leads people to become dehydrated is the belief that tea, coffee, alcohol, and soft drinks are suitable and equal substitutes for natural water. Actually, they contain dehydrating agents, which not only encourage water loss through kidneys, lungs, skin, and GI system, but they take some water from body reserves with it. In fact, Chronic Fatigue Syndrome has been related to drinking excessive amounts of caffeinated beverages because it depletes the energy molecule (ATP) stores in the brain and the body.

In *The Choice Is Clear,* Dr. Allen E. Banik explains how water functions in the body, the effects of pollutants in drinking water sources and their contribution to disease, and how to obtain pure water.   But, briefly, to help you determine if your glass is half-empty or half full, here are a few guidelines to assist in defining what we are calling "water" these days.

Hard water (public water systems) is believed by many to be our greatest health enemy. Hard 'tap' water can contain viruses, bacteria, chemicals, and many other harmful inorganic minerals and chemicals.   These inorganic minerals obtained from the air and ground cannot be used by the body unless they are changed to organic minerals, the only form our body can use. Consequently, these minerals may collect in different parts of our bodies, causing arthritis, constipation, gout, varicose veins, emphysema, and glaucoma.   Research shows that in an individual who drinks a gallon of hard water each day, is drinking up to 450 glasses of mineral solids during their life span, particles of which our body must remove.

Distilled water is called the "purest kind of water," the only kind that can be taken into the body without causing damage to the tissues. All minerals (the good and the bad) are removed, so supplementation of a good organic mineral formula is a good idea.

Filtered water is effective in eliminating chlorine, but bacteria and viruses easily pass through the filters.   The matter that collects at the bottom of the filter can also harbor bacteria, contaminating the water all over again.

Bottled water is convenient and for the most part is free of chemicals, but not strictly regulated for safety, so can contain bacteria. The most harmful aspect of bottled water, however, is the possible leaching of the plastic from the bottle into the water, especially if it has been in a warm storage place.

Before we judge whose water is good, whose is not, it is best to contact the Environmental Protection Agency to inquire about testing your water.

* * *

SLEEPING IN A TOXIC BEDROOM

Safe-and-sound and snuggled under the covers? Tucked in for the night on a firm mattress, clean sheets, and a comfy pillow and you are all set for eight hours of blissful sleep. Right? Maybe not.

Health conditions such as memory loss, headaches, depression, and itchy eyes can arise from exposure to a seemingly innocent bedroom environment. Most mattresses and pillows, for example, are filled with chemical-drenched synthetic fibers such as polyurethane foam that release chemicals into the air for years, causing headaches and nausea, and can even lead to multiple chemical sensitivities (MCS), a condition that stems from exposure to toxic chemicals and results in a myriad of crippling symptoms.

Microscopic dust mites (and their allergenic fecal matter) frequently infest mattresses pillow, and carpeting, leading to respiratory problems including coughing and sinus congestion. And the results of exposure to electromagnetic fields, or EMFs, which can be emitted from your alarm clock, have been linked to cancer.

Making your bedroom a safer, healthier, and more restful place may require attention to several different areas. Polyester sheets are actually soft thermoplastic, which is made from petrochemicals. The most harmful bed linens you can buy are polyester "no-iron" and wrinkle-resistant sheets, since not only are they made from petrochemicals, but also are often treated with a formaldehyde resin finish. This finish is permanent and cannot be removed from the fiber. Unfortunately, fabrics coated with formaldehyde will release gases for life. It is thought that up to a fifth of the general population may be sensitive to formaldehyde gases, even at very low concentrations.

Symptoms of formaldehyde sensitivity include tiredness and insomnia, coughing, irritation of throat and eyes, headaches, nausea, and nosebleeds. Formaldehyde is also a suspected carcinogen (causer-causing agent). Look for sheets made from unbleached cotton, cotton flannel, or linen. Always wash bed linens before using them to eliminate any manufacturing or shipping fine particles.

More trouble may be found in mattresses and pillows, most of them being stuffed with polyurethane foam, which can cause respiratory problems as well as skin and eye irritation, and because they can harbor dust mites. The mattress foam can also release toluene diisoyanate, a chemical that can cause severe lung problems. The highest concentrations of these hazardous chemicals are released during the first few years of the mattress's life. Cotton mattresses are

48

much better, if you can find them, or consider using cotton mattress pads and mattress covers. A tightly woven cotton mattress or pillow covers (not treated with formaldehyde) can seal in dust mite fecal matter, eliminating allergic reactions to those that may be living in your mattress and pillows.

Cotton-filled pillows are recommended as a better alternative to chemical-drenched polyester foam.

Being snug-as-a-bug-in-a-rug may not be as good as it sounds, as dirty carpet from elements brought into the bedroom from feet, shoes, or boots also create a breeding ground for dust mites. Not only are mites toxic to our lungs, but also the gases given off from the layers of synthetic fabrics, starting with the carpet padding. These fumes are capable of producing burning eyes, chills and fever, memory loss, blurred vision, and depression.

The hundreds of toxic gases coming from new carpeting have been reported to cause illness in both children and adults and are responsible for the "new carpet smell."

As with mattresses, the greatest quantities of gases are emitted in the first five years of the carpet's life. Certainly, hard wood floors are easily cleaned and less likely to retain toxic components. Rugs made of natural cotton, jute, and cotton-coils are also good health alternatives.

New furniture, as well, can emit dangerous levels of gases from veneered particleboard, whereas older or antique furniture that are fifty or more years no longer are guilty of this.

Getting the toxins out of the bedroom will help us awake with the renewed health and vitality that a good night's sleep is designed to provide…a state of health that some of us are, unfortunately, still only dreaming about.

* * *

Twenty Ways to Love Your Liver

Ever feel like you have to keep poisoning yourself just to stay alive?

Strange as it sounds, the coffee we drink to wake up, the drugs we take to get "well", the artificial sweeteners we use to reduce calories, and the junk food we grab to stave off starvation are all poisoning us.

Over time, these toxins begin to accumulate in your body, creating a higher and higher hurdle required of our health to mount in order for us to stay optimally healthy. The mere act of "living," adds its own list of toxic accumulation, especially if we eat, drink, or breath in a toxic environment.

One of the goals of naturopathic medicine is to help people identity their sources of toxins, develop a plan to remove them, and then lend help and support as they begin to address the process of clearing their toxic buildup. The term most often used for this process is "detoxification." Disorders related to toxic overload include: fatigue, pain, headaches, depression, intestinal distress, allergies, arteriolosclerosis, inflammatory joint disease, and more.

Some detox programs, often promoted by those who are not medically trained to monitor a safe and effective plan, manage only to "stir up" poisons in people, adding to their ill health, not helping. The error that is made in such plans, is that of leaving out the first step – that of opening the "organs of elimination." Unless these organs are clear and ready to receive the toxins that are being identified in the body, and about to be eliminated, toxins merely flow from one area to the other, often leaving a person feeling more fatigued, "flu-ish", and sometimes in dangerously worse health.

Organs to "open" so that poisons can exit the body are the kidneys, the colon, the lungs, the skin, and the liver. Each body system has a simple, yet effective method of clearing and refreshing itself, readying itself for its job of detoxifying the body. But each systems must be "up and running" for the best and safest benefit from detoxification.

Of special importance to the optimal health of the body, is the health of the liver. Weighing about four pounds, the liver is the largest organ in the body and the only internal organ that many say will regenerate itself, given proper support, if it is damaged or diseased.

The liver has many functions, making it perhaps the most important organ in the body, aside from the brain and heart. It secretes bile needed to digest fats, assists in the absorption of some

50

vitamins, helps in the metabolizing of fat to produce energy, participates in the regulation of blood sugar, helps with thyroid function, and is active in detoxification (removal) of poisons from the body, including pharmaceutical drugs.

With decreased liver function, good organ health throughout the body is lessened, metabolism decreases causing fatigue and weight gain, digestion is impaired creating pain and bowel dysfunction, vitamins throughout the body become deficient, the brain develops "brain fog", and the skin becomes unhealthy and starts "breaking out." In essence, the body becomes a cesspool of toxic waste and impaired function.

The main culprits contributing to liver disease and toxicity are the buildup over time of alcohol, insecticide and pesticide residues, ammonia as a by-product of protein (meat) digestion, and recreational, over-the-counter, and pharmaceutical drugs. Common day-to-day interactions with the environment like new carpeting, "bathing" in gasoline, traffic fumes, second-hand cigarette smoke, and paint fumes from newly painted rooms also contribute to liver toxicity. Normal processes within the body, called metabolic by-products, are being produced continually giving the liver toxins to get rid of, even without the onslaught of outside influences.

One of the best supportive options for good liver health is the use of the herb, milk thistle (*silymarin*). Milk thistle contains some of the most potent liver-protecting natural substances known. Research shows that it stimulates the production of new liver cells and prevents formation of damaging chemicals that encourage liver damage. Milk thistle is also good for the kidneys, the colon, the skin, and the immune system, making it an excellent therapeutic for improved functioning of all the organs of elimination, given the correct dosage from a good product resource.

Although treatment plans are always specific to each person, general recommendations for good liver health for most everyone include: Drink freshly prepared vegetable juices including beets and carrots, and other *fresh* "green" drinks. Avoid heavy, constipating foods. Be sure your diet has sufficient amounts of bulk and fiber. Avoid the toxins in processed and packaged foods. Avoid a diet high in fat, cooked oils, sugars, and white flour products. Do not overeat. Overeating creates too much work for the liver, causing liver fatigue.

Remember, the toxins that you put in your body by way of eating, drinking, or breathing your body systems must deal with. Listen to what your body is telling you. You *know* when it is time to quit overloading your liver with poisons. Make the right choices, and optimal health is your reward.

* * *

MEN'S HEALTH

MEN'S HEALTH: THE POWER OF SAW PALMETTO

Men, as well as women, need all the health tools they can get. And, it has been said that a job becomes easiest when the right tool is used. When it comes to protecting men's prostate, the more "tools" they can get, the easier it will be to stay healthy.

You may be surprised to know that the tool you may need may not be found in the tool shed. This 'saw' comes from the earth; it is saw palmetto (*Serenoa repens*).

The value of naturopathic medicine is that we can draw from health tools from every medical system in the world: those of Europe, India, China, and more. Originally, the American Indian consumed saw palmetto berries as part of their diet. Today, supported by research from European clinical study discoveries, we know that the greatest therapeutic benefit from saw palmetto is in treating the prostate for BPH (Benign Prostatic Hypertrophy). A standardized extract of the fat-soluble part of the berries has shown remarkably consistent pharmacological effects, showing no side effects through toxicology studies in animals.

BPH is thought to be caused when testosterone levels build up in the prostate. Within the prostate, testosterone is converted into an even more potent compound call dihydrotestosterone (DHT). This compound causes cells to multiply excessively, eventually leading to prostate enlargement (most commonly after the age of 50), and sometimes cancer.

Studies have shown the oils in the berries prevent the conversion of testosterone to DHT and help to increase the breakdown and excretion of existing dihydrotestosterone in the prostate gland. Clinical evidence and verification from imaging and physical exams, confirms that another natural nutrient, zinc, may reduce the size of the prostate and decrease related symptoms in most patients. Together, in their proper dosages, saw palmetto and zinc have shown dramatic results for prostate inflammation and enlargement, and BPH prevention.

Given the fact that each year, over $1 billion is spent on hospital care and surgery for this condition, the standardized extract of saw palmetto berries may offer an effective alternative to surgery.

But buyer beware. Work with a doctor who is up on the latest saw palmetto research, to receive the proper amounts needed for your individual requirement. Accurate dosage is vital for optimal results, as is a complete review of current health issues and past medical history before treatment begins. The brand is also important. Many discount (cheap) "over-the-counter" supplements do not contain "active" ingredients that our body actually utilizes.

The best source of saw palmetto will come from a research company or medical laboratory. Do not waste your money, or your health, by taking the wrong supplement.

This year for Father's Day, ask for a tool. But ask for a 'health tool', so you can give back to your family what they deserve...a healthy you.

* * *

The "Men" in Menopause

We've all heard of menopause, a condition from which a woman often suffers as a result of female hormone deficiencies. But who has heard of male menopause? Actually, the medical term is "adropause". The name reflects a condition of deficiency of androgen hormones, the testosterone and DHEA hormones that gives that "get-up-and-go" to the male. And, in fact, andropause is of real concern to many an unconfessing male.

There often are overlapping causes for concern, as the man begins to see his mind (and body) slip into andropause. His physical changes may be psychologically depressing, as often happens with women during menopause. Such awareness of deteriorating physical health can affect a man's self-esteem, common responses to testosterone deficiency. When a man has hormonal disturbances that interfere with his sexual function and physical endurance, the resulting feelings of loss and depression can cause an andropausal condition, symptoms also common to many women over 45.

Testosterone deficiency is a physical abnormality. The hormone, which is also present in smaller amounts in women, is needed for the normal functioning of the nervous and muscular system, to delay bone demineralization, and to maintain a feeling of well-being and sexuality. Andropause is a mental reaction to the symptoms from the decline in testosterone, often causing unhappiness and concern.

Although still uncertain whether male menopause is a result of hormone deficiency or a psychological condition because of the declining physical effects, there are ways to replace that which may have been lost, be it hormone replacement or from other natural help resources.

The onset of andropause is most common between the ages of forty and sixty, but most frequently appears in the late fifties when a man realizes his life is more than half over. Common physical symptoms which may bring about the depression of andropause include: muscle weakness and less endurance, increase or decrease in weight with changes in appetite, less body hair, and impairment of sexual function.

Often caused by testosterone deficiency, an accurate hormone level can be determined by simple lab tests, through either blood (doctor's office) or saliva (home test).

What are the solutions to a declining testosterone level? According to Jonathan Wright, MD, "For restoring sexuality and the diverse aspects of men's health known to deteriorate with age natural testosterone, as well as specific vitamins, amino acids, and herbal and botanical products are demonstrably more effective and safer in the human body than any synthetic hormone or pharmaceutical drugs."

As with commonly prescribed estrogens, synthetic hormones that masquerade as natural hormones are similar in molecular structure, but are never exactly the same as the natural molecule. Unfortunately, because drug molecules are different, the body treats them differently, which usually leads to adverse and even dangerous side effects. As is the case with synthetic testosterone, they can be liver damage, blood clots, reducing the "good" cholesterol (HDL), and increasing the "bad" (LDL).

By working with a licensed doctor, who will take a detailed medical history first, men interested in natural testosterone replacement can select from applications of creams, gels, patches, and under-the-tongue (sublingual) tablets. Pills that are swallowed are less desirable and not as effective, as they must pass through the liver, leaving virtually none of its active hormone in the body. By going directly into the blood stream, as with a gel, cream, or a sublingual form, the liver can be by-passed, providing a useable amount of biologically active hormone. Always consider any potential side effects or new research on this subject before deciding.

For those not prone to replace natural testosterone, there are many ways to boost the body's own ability to overcome andropause. The amino acid, L-arginine, has been found to raise levels of nitric oxide in the body. This is the molecule that facilitates increased blood flow and engorgement of the penis; in other words, encourages a strong erection. Simply explained, the L-arginine supplies the nitrogen needed to build the "N" of NO (nitric oxide), a safe and natural way of overcoming the effects of testosterone deficiency.

Another important hormone for maintaining a youthful virility, and assisting with weight management, is growth hormone. It drops drastically as men (and women) grow older. Adding an ample supply to the diet (in supplemental pill or powder form) of the amino acid proteins - glutamine, lysine, and arginine - can often help boost human growth hormone levels by assisting its natural production in the body.

Other botanical (plant) resources for male menopause are many, but a few of my favorites are these: *Panax ginseng* is great for increasing physical endurance, reducing blood pressure, lowering cholesterol, and enhancing fertility and libido. It also may increase the erectile effects of nitric oxide as discussed above.

Muira puama is a shrub that grows in the Amazon region of Brazil. Studies have revealed that it, too, has been shown to be a natural treatment for men with sexual disorders, a common symptom of andropause.

Gingko biloba, another botanical remedy prominent in Asia and the U.S, is known for increasing blood flow to areas of the body described as "peripheral." That is why it is good for brain, feet and toes, and other parts where good blood flow is appreciated.

Not to go unmentioned is the concern over too much testosterone and the self-dosing of androgens-producing supplements, such as DHEA (not to be confused with the essential fatty acid, DHA). This can be avoided by obtaining simple saliva lab tests results of DHEA and testosterone, and checking the results for abnormally high levels, as too much of a good thing is not a good thing. DHEA is the pre-cursor to testosterone, and while adequate levels of DHEA can be beneficial, excessively high levels over months or years can alter other levels of hormones. Chronically elevated levels of androgen hormones might encourage prostate cancer, just as inappropriately prescribed estrogen for women who are already estrogen-excessive can also be harmful.

Whether they outright admit it or not, men are beginning to pause and take second looks at themselves in the mirror, a habit we once thought was reserved for women.

With this growing concern over male hormone deficiency and stamina preservation, one wonders if the word 'men-o-pause', was actually meant for men all along.

* * *

WOMEN'S HEALTH

Hormone Study: Wake Up Call to Women

A wake-up call for women has sounded. The message is clear. The warnings are out. The published results of a study found that not only does synthetic hormone replacement therapy (HRT) not prevent heart disease, that they may in fact actually cause it. Incidences in stroke and breast cancer were also increased in test subjects taking Prempro® (a combination of Premarin and Progestin).

Anyone who claims, "I will take my chances," and continues to take them without careful thought, has clearly not had a close encounter of the cancer-kind yet.

According to the *Natural Medicines Comprehensive Database* compiled by a group of registered pharmacists, synthetic estrogens including Premarin®, Ogen®, Estrace®, Estratab®, Cenestin®, Prempro®, Premphase®, and oral contraceptives containing estrogen can cause nutritional depletions of vitamin B6 and B12. Oral contraceptives are especially B vitamin depletors, as they lower levels of folic acid as well. These nutrients are needed to protect the heart from high homocysteine levels. With high levels of this amino acid, heart problems increase, a reason for those taking synthetic estrogens to supplement for preventative protection.

However, what about those women who have taken estrogens, and not re-supplied their B6, B12, and folic acid deficiencies? Your conclusion is the same as mine, higher incidences of heart disease, the number one killer of women today. That makes an interesting connection no one is making.

Estrogens also deplete us of magnesium, an important mineral that is essential for proper calcium absorption into the bones. Without the balance of magnesium, most supplemental calcium is not absorbed into the bones, causing dangerously high levels of calcium to circulate through blood vessels in the body. "Calcification" of the arteries may result. In the end, more heart disease, not to mention increased bone loss (osteoporosis) without magnesium.

Most conventional medical doctors are not trained to look for nutritional deficiencies that result from drugs and common over-the-counter medications, including those occurring from conventional hormone replacement therapy. Only those with special interests in this field taking time to research this new area of medicine of drug-induced nutrient depletions will include it in their patient treatment plan. Unfortunately, as the study reveals, the deficiencies being caused by conventional hormone replacements (and some calcium supplements) may have with years of use actually caused women's hearts more harm than good.

Medical science is constantly advancing to new areas and as such, increased information is available to those who seek it. Often there is more research than there is time in a day to grasp it all. Consequently, information regarding nutritional deficiencies from prescription drugs is slow to filter through the patient population.

But if the issues regarding key nutrient deficiencies by synthetic hormones are not brought up, heart disease in women will continue to rise. Research is showing that women with a family medical history of heart disease and breast cancer should not take synthetic estrogens for more than a brief time. If on the other hand, they want to take their chances, they should supplement with magnesium and B vitamins (including folic acid) to protect their hearts from the damage the depletions may be creating.

But, you argue, my doctor says my Premarin® is "natural." Yes, equine estrogens (horse urine) used in Premarin® and Prempro® are called "natural" by many doctors and also by the company who makes these prescription drugs. (They use the urine obtained from pregnant horses in horse "farms" created specifically to serve this purpose, farms with no use for the mare's offspring.)

However, according to Christianne Northrup, MD, nationally-known board certified doctor of obstetrics and gynecology, "Studies have shown that when Premarin is metabolized in the human body, its breakdown products are biologically stronger and therefore potentially more apt to promote cancer, than the breakdown products of bio-identical estrogens." Current research is now concluding what many have been saying all along, "Conjugated equine estrogens can be harmful to women's health."

Instead of stressing over what will happen if the hormones are discontinued, I say to those women, ask yourself what may happen if you continue to take them. The recent study on Prempro® was quickly stopped because researchers were finding too many adverse effects in their test subjects to warrant continuing the study with safety. Specifically increases in blood clots, gallbladder disease, strokes, heart attacks, and breast cancer were shown to occur after just a few years of synthetic hormone use.

Women have been lead to believe for decades that their long-term health depended upon them taking Premarin® and Prempro®, as doctors prescribed them as if they were vitamins. Now, with the clinical studies indicating the opposite, they are forced to look at health solutions they (and their doctors) have long forgotten.

I advise, support the heart with exercise and heart healthy nutrients (especially if they have been depleted from hormone use), eat calcium-rich foods or supplement with the proper blend of calcium, magnesium, and vitamin D3 for continued bone health, add the elements that help prevent Alzheimer's, support the systems that produce our own supply of hormones, and manage any excessive stress that could put you into an early grave.

If you are bothered with menopausal symptoms and need a temporary management "bridge", consider a bio-identical hormone replacement for a short time (one that matches the molecule of that of the human female body) until these uncomfortable symptoms subside. Doctors can prescribe these from their choices of bio-identical hormone selections if a woman requests it.

Do not panic, but do be concerned. This is not an issue to be dismissed, but one to address or you may be traveling down a road that recent research is now clearly advising against.

This is your wake up call. Take your chances if you choose to, but do so as an informed, responsible, adult woman.

* * *

The important thing is to not stop questioning.

ALBERT EINSTEIN
1879 - 1955

THE EXPERTS SPEAK ON ESTROGEN

The truth is, more and more women are asking their doctors to take them off their synthetic hormones.

Their questions still arise, however, regarding what is safe, what is protective, and what is to be more closely monitored. In order to help them answer their questions, I have turned to my favorite medical experts to see what they say.

In addition, although I have my own opinions on the subject, and I still believe we each need to do our own research and consult with our doctors, I will let them speak for me this time. In so doing, I will try to present a concise assessment of what they are currently saying to women these days. So be prepared to be shocked, even horrified, as we begin.

Jonathan Wright, MD, reminds us that, "Premarin®" is horse urine. It is derived from the urine of pregnant mares, hence its name. (*Pre*gnant *Mar*e's Ur*ine*) Replacing human estrogens with horse estrogens may be asking for trouble." He continues to explain, "Those alien horse urine estrogens (equilin) that are currently being prescribed, are not handled very well by the human body."

"As a result," Dr. Wright says, "Premarin® can produce 'estrogenic effects' which are much more potent and longer lasting than those produced by natural human estrogens." He wonders why doctors do not more often use these natural-to-human estrogens. Premarin® is a patented pill (and cream), a big-business prescription often covered by insurance, whereas, natural estrogens formulated in dosages designed specifically to replace only deficiencies, are usually not covered.

"Premarin® is widely considered by physicians to be a 'natural' hormone product, because it is derived from horse urine, and is even described as 'natural' in the package insert. But when placed in the human body, the hormones in Premarin® are as foreign as any synthetic drug," Dr. Wright says.

Echoing Dr. Wright's sentiments, Dr. Joel Hargrove, medical director of the Menopause Center at Vanderbilt University Medical Center in Tennessee, says, "Premarin® is a natural hormone if your native food is hay."

Premarin®'s manufacturer's package insert confirms the contents as being that of horse urine, and described its capsules as also containing Yellow Dye No. 10, Blue No. 1, Blue No. 2, Red No. 27, Red No. 40, Red No. 7, among others.

Not to be ignored is the bold print warning in the first paragraph of the package insert which say, "Estrogens have been reported to increase the risk of endometrial carcinoma in postmenopausal women," and advises later in the Premarin® printout, that if you use estrogen, in order to reduce risk of estrogen use, you and your doctor should re-evaluate whether or not you still need estrogens at least every six months.

Dr. John Lee, MD, promotes the health benefits of another bio-identical hormone, natural progesterone, as opposed to the synthetic Provera® (medroxyprogesterone). He says, "It is my belief that our doctors need to be re-educated in the realities of their female patients' hormone matters."

Casting doubt on the use of synthetic estrogen, board-certified ob-gyn and author, Christianne Northrup, MD, says regarding Premarin®, "Equine (horse) estrogens are often associated with side effects such as headaches, bloating, and sore breasts. A host of studies have shown that breakdown products from Premarin® are very strong and can produce DNA changes that are carcinogenic (cancer-causing) in tissue."

"Given this," she continues, "it's no wonder that the incidence of breast cancer statistically increases when women are on this drug. In contrast, the metabolic breakdown products of bio-identical (natural) estrogens are biologically weaker, so their effects on tissue do not last as long." She admits, however, that more long-term studies are needed."

Dr. Northrup advises that women's hormone levels be measured by saliva tests to determine their levels of estrogen before they begin any hormone replacement. Often times, symptoms are a result of low progesterone, not low estrogen. By automatically supplementing estrogen without first confirming a deficiency, symptoms of estrogen excess can occur. This can result, however, from either too much synthetic or natural estrogen.

Can we avoid replacing estrogen after menopause and still have healthy hearts and bones, many ask? Although research still leans toward estrogens as being beneficial for the heart and bones, many authorities are emphasizing instead the contributions that diet and exercise have on cardiovascular and bone health, thereby eliminating the harm that synthetic estrogen use many cause.

It seems to a growing number of medical doctors that we have forgotten the basics of preventive care, and are instead counting too heavily on this synthetic drug to do the job. Natural health spokesman, Andrew Weil, MD, agrees, saying, "I think the current wave of enthusiasm for this hormone blinds us to its possible hazards, especially on increase cancer risks."

What happened to exercise and restricted dietary saturated fats as key to a healthy heart? Where is the list of bone-building nutrients upon which we are to focus for continued bone strength? If animal estrogens are so good for heart and bone health, as we are so often told, perhaps we will soon find them fortifying our milk and meats, at a store near you, so that even our kids may benefit.

But even scarier though, perhaps they already are.

* * *

THE PROS OF PROGESTERONE

In the last chapter, we discussed estrogen and how it can help or hurt postmenopausal women, working especially well for hot flashes and night sweats, common symptoms of "estrogen deficiency." What most women do not know, however, is that synthetic estrogen supplementation can often be avoided and women can still eliminate their bothersome symptoms with supplementation of natural progesterone.

Dr. John Lee, family practice MD, was one of the first to recommend progesterone cream to his patients in the late 1970s. He says in his book, *What Your Doctor May Not Tell You about Menopause*, "Because progesterone is a biochemical precursor to estrogen in the body, it alone is often sufficient to restore estrogen levels to normal."

He cautions us about the use of synthetic progestin (Provera®), saying, "We have a widespread misconception among American doctors that natural progesterone has the same side effects as the progestins – an error that is dramatically affecting the health and well-being of millions of American women." He continues to explain that natural progesterone, when used in amounts no greater than what the body should be making, has no known side effects, while the synthetic progestins have many.

That list of precautions and adverse reactions from medroxyprogesterone acetate (synthetic progesterone), as described in the *Physicians' Desk Reference (PDR)*, include "breakthrough bleeding, spotting, change in menstrual flow, acne, alopecia (hair loss), insomnia, migraines, asthma, and mental depression to name a few. (Women with undiagnosed vaginal bleeding should not take synthetic progestins, Dr. Lee says.)

Provera®, when taken with estrogens, has been observed to cause rise in blood pressure, water retention, headaches, dizziness, fatigue, loss of scalp hair, urinary tract infections, change in sex drive, and others, Dr. Lee describes.

In comparison, natural progesterone protects against endometrial and breast cancer (which synthetic estrogens may contribute to causing), improves sleep patterns, improves new bone formation, prevents further hair loss, and helps normalize cholesterol, says Dr. Lee.

According to Jonathan V. Wright, MD, "Although much evidence suggests that estrogen replacement helps reduce the risks associated with heart disease, new data confirms that the common practice of taking the synthetic progestin, Provera®, along with estrogen to minimize the risk of endometrial cancer may be increasing women's risk of suffering a heart attack to an unacceptable level. Natural progesterone, however, provides cancer protection but carries no such risk."

In his book *Natural Hormone Replacement*, Dr. Wright quotes one researcher of a British study who said, "In terms of heart disease protection, Provera® is worse than no treatment at all."

Neither estrogens nor progestins should be considered as automatic one-a-day supplements for every woman after menopause, as many doctors suggest. The experts agree, saying treat the patient as symptoms and risk factors require for as long as symptoms persist.

Some doctors do not understand the pros of progesterone, and do not offer it to their patients who have had hysterectomies, saying that there is no reason to prescribe it, despite the long list of benefits studies have indicated. Dr. Christianne Northrup, MD, says, "Progesterone also effects brain function. It produces a sense of calmness, and its sedating, anti-anxiety effect helps promote rejuvenated sleep." She, too, never recommends any hormone replacement therapies that employ synthetic progestins, which she feels actually causes or exaggerates many symptoms.

After assessing accurate levels of progesterone through saliva testing, Dr. Northrup recommends bio-identical resources (same molecule as is the human molecule) of progesterone in cream or pill form, but cautions using formulas containing wild yam. "The problem is," Dr. Northrup says, "Yam contains only a progesterone precursor, which remains inactive when it is absorbed through the skin. Consequently, yam creams don't provide the documented benefits of progesterone."

Dr. Northrup points out that most studies conducted on hormone replacement have been done using, synthetic, not bio-identical hormones. She says we urgently need long-term studies on the natural, bio-identical, individualized hormone replacement, in order to provide adequate guidance to women and their physicians. "But given the politics of medicine and research, including the fact that bio-identical hormones cannot be patented," she says, "we're not likely to have these studies for a long time to come."

That will put many women on hold for longer they may be willing to wait. Why don't more doctors recommend natural hormones over synthetics? Certainly, proper training on natural hormone replacement is essential, but never included in conventional medical curriculums. Also essential is a doctor's interest and time necessary to devote to studying the recent research, as well as wanting to network with other physicians who are also not bound strictly what their drug reps offer.

From the patient's perspective, a financial investment into their own health is often necessary, since an individualized hormone consultation, testing, and then customized formulation is often not covered by insurance, unless ordered by their primary care physician for menopausal symptoms. But without their extra study on natural hormones, and the lack of sufficient studies, doctors will hesitate to stray from the established "standard of care" to prescribe natural hormone replacement, despite the growing number of requests from their patients.

It is hard to blame either side, as both doctors and women want the greatest safety and symptomatic relief that hormone replacement can offer. However, nothing ventured is nothing gained. And times, they are a-changin'.

* * *

DIGESTIVE SYSTEM

A Little Bacteria on the Side, Please

In a world of antibiotics, is there such a thing as an equal and opposite probiotic? Yes. And if you have unexplained digestive problems including gas, bloating, and diarrhea, then this may be the missing piece of information that could help turn your health around.

The word "probiotic" comes from two Greek words meaning "for life" and refers to organisms such as beneficial bacteria, which contribute to the health and balance of the intestinal tract. They benefit us by keeping the balance of what has essentially become a barren wasteland of literally no bacteria, often times after antibiotic use. Most of us have heard a reference to lactobacillus acidophilus, since it is found in many brands of yogurts. This is just one of many forms of probiotics that will benefit our health.

When we refer to bacteria, we are programmed to think of eliminating them as quickly as possible for fear of infection. Very little information has been distributed about the beneficial effects of some strains of bacteria. If you have not heard about probiotics before today, at least now you now have a little something to chew on.

Factors which cause an imbalance in these helpful microscopic beings are sugary diets, stress levels, and as we've said, the over-use of antibiotics. Almost any antibiotic given by mouth can severely alter the balance and pattern of the intestinal flora. The reduction in total populations of the flora caused by antibiotics can be dramatic. Unfortunately, the ecological vacuum created by the indiscriminate slaughter of friendly bacteria is often rapidly filled by potentially pathogenic (disease causing) microorganisms.

Clostridium difficile, a notorious opportunistic bacteria which populates the large intestine during treatment with antibiotics, especially ampicillin, has been reported to destroy the surface of the colon, producing ulcerations and consequent symptoms of bloody diarrhea, pain, and unhealthy weight loss. *Candida albicans* deserves mention, since a wide range of symptoms are possible as a result of its rapid overgrowth after antibiotic treatment. Researchers have shown that symptoms such as fatigue, gas and bloating, constipation or diarrhea, allergies, and depression can be related to yeast overgrowth in the colon, after an antibiotic treatment has made more room for the yeast to grow. (Remember, antibiotics only kill bacteria, not viruses, or yeast.)

Dysbiosis, the alteration for the worse of the ecology of the digestive tract, has been shown to be at the very forefront of causes of major and destructive diseases. Probiotics, the restoration by safe supplementation and diet of this intestinal ecosystem, offers a solution for dysbiosis. Think of replanting flowers and trees to prevent overgrowth of weeds in a once beautifully populated garden that was burned out by a fire and you will understand the basic concept of taking probiotics after antibiotic therapy.

Although eating yogurt is the probiotic therapy most doctors recommend, don't forget that many of us do not tolerate dairy, a condition that could cause the very symptoms we are trying to avoid. I prefer to supplement a refrigerated resource in pill or powder form to get the highest dosage possible without the added dairy or, even worse, the sugars found in yogurt.

It is a strange concept, indeed, that we would actually want to ingest living bacteria. Nevertheless, whether you can swallow the idea or not, both science and nature agree that bacteria that promotes good health and prevents those unexpected runs to the bathroom could not be that bad after all.

* * *

IRRITABLE BOWEL: A PROCESS OF ELIMINATION

Is your digestive system ill and irritable with you? Are you developing a close, personal relationship with your bathroom toilet? If so, you may have what many have called Irritable Bowel Syndrome (IBS).

This is a common condition, affecting 10-20% of all American adults and is the most common gastrointestinal complaint even though many never seek the help of a physician. Varieties of symptoms are present including: constipation alternating with diarrhea (the most common pattern), abdominal pain, gas, bloating, secretions of colon mucous, nausea, and sometimes accompanied by varying degrees of anxiety or depression.

The causes of IBS are not completely clear, but dietary factors, plus psychological factors, have been linked to this condition. It can significantly restrict one's lifestyle, making it the second most common reason for missing work, next to the common cold.

A change in one's diet can often be curative in IBS. Dietary fiber and complex carbohydrates (foods found in their whole form that have not been refined) are useful in normalizing bowel function. People with diarrhea may be at first aggravated with the initial introduction of dietary fiber, such as the raw foods in salads. The best types of fiber to include are called water-soluble found in vegetables, fruits, oat bran, beans and peas, and psyllium seed powder. Wheat and other grains are an excellent form of fiber but very often can cause allergic reactions.

Research shows a high correlation between people with IBS and single or multi food intolerances. It is important to identify these causes and eliminate the offending sources. The best test to determine these involves a program of a 6-week elimination diet. This is a diet which leaves out the common foods usually thought to aggravate and irritate bowels. After 6 weeks, foods are reintroduced one at a time every 3 days. If symptoms worsen or return, that food should not be eaten again.

Most people with IBS complain of some mental/emotional factors such as insomnia, fatigue, and anxiety. Increased contractions of the colon have been shown to occur in people with IBS in response to stressful situations, including worry about present or future events, often triggering IBS symptoms. Learning stress modification techniques can alter abnormal digestive reactions. If we don't react with alarm to a situation, our body doesn't sense it as stressful.

Various botanical and nutritional supplements are helpful in the treatment of IBS. Peppermint oil has been used to inhibit GI contractions and relieve abdominal pain and gas. Enteric-coated peppermint oil capsules deliver the oil to the small intestine and bypass the stomach. Other botanicals that act to decrease the symptoms are chamomile, slippery elm, lemon balm, and rosemary in tea, tincture, or capsule form. Nutritional supplements such as glutamine, beta-carotene, and zinc help in the healing of the intestinal wall lining, important in the treatment of IBS. Consult a nutritionally licensed physician for safe and effective dosages, as they will take your complete medical history into account before making recommendations.

Perhaps most important in the symptomatic relief is food choices. Here is a list of foods to avoid: cabbage family foods (especially broccoli, Brussels sprouts, and cauliflower), wheat, corn, dairy products, citrus fruits, and chocolate, spicy foods, alcohol, cheese, vinegar, coffee and black tea, pork, and sugar and sugar deserts.

You will find that sugar is everywhere. If you want to truly avoid sugars to determine if your symptoms will improve, check labels for glucose, sucrose, malt, maltose, corn syrup, fructose, brown sugar, honey, maple syrup, molasses, lactose, and sorbitol. If you find that sugars are your problem, it is well worth your health to eliminate them. In addition, if you feel worse after eating sugars, seriously consider candida overgrowth as a contributing factor.

Many people are 'fructose-sensitive' so search for a list of high-fructose foods and avoid. I have seen merely implementing this one step has solved many IBS conditions.

Beneficial foods include: steamed or baked vegetables of all kinds, split peas, lentils, potatoes, brown rice, oatmeal, kidney beans, and oat bran.

Low-fat, high-fiber diets are best, although each person has their own set of food sensitivities. Eat small meals, and chew foods well. If you want to add fiber supplement, try psyllium seeds or husks, but follow it with adequate water intake.

Antibiotics are a well-known cause of temporary diarrhea and other GI problems, and steroid medications can also affect the balance of flora. The good flora is eliminated, especially in people who are on repeated doses of antibiotics, which allow other harmful microbes to dominate the intestinal tract. Acidophilus and bifidobacteria supplements (from a refrigerated resource) can help restore intestinal balance and help to reduce GI complaints.

Remember that both diet and stress can be factors in how much time you have to spend in the bathroom. It is not necessarily what you are eating, though, that is causing the problem, but what is eating you.

* * *

IMMUNE SYSTEM

Catch the Cold Before it Catches You

If you are one of the lucky ones who have not gotten sick this year, good for you. The wellness program to which you committed earlier in the year has richly rewarded you.

If, on the other hand, the bug has bitten you, time to get back on top of health and recommit to being well through the next few months, especially if you have partaken in the sugary treats as far back as Halloween. Remember, sugar lessens the power of your immune system to fight disease, so time to eliminate that "food group" from your cabinets, freezers, and shopping list.

Begin to follow these supplement and lifestyle recommendations immediately to keep your immune system strong. Remember, allergy season is just around the corner.

- Take 500 mg of vitamin C with bioflavonoids two times a day, plus 15 milligrams of zinc once or twice times a day. Take these in "divided doses," not all at once. You may take them together with food.

- Pour supplements into the lid, and then throw them into your mouth (followed by water). Do not pour them into your hands, and put your hands to your mouth. Manufacturers take great care in not contaminating your supplements. Don't you contaminate them by touching them!

- Keep neck, throat, arms, and feet covered and warm to prevent "wind chill."

- Keep hands washed and be aware of putting hands to eyes, nose, and mouth. These are entry points for bacteria.

- Don't eat "public food." This is food you may find at parties, hotel lobbies, or public buffets that others may have touched, sneezed on, or coughed on and have been contaminated.

- Don't lick your fingers to turn pages. Again, bacteria are abundant on hands, even after you wash them.

- Change your toothbrush frequently.

- Don't breathe through your mouth in cold weather; breathe through your nose.

- Don't eat sugar; it depletes your immune system and feeds bacteria.

- Avoid people who are coughing and sneezing. Don't shake too many hands, as they may have just sneezed into them.

- Drink lots of pure water and increase consumption of nutritious foods.

- Avoid too much stress; stress runs down your immune system and depletes the vitamin C stores in your body.

- Avoid crowds.

* * *

Dr. Yerby's Cold and Flu Protocol:

Prevention, usually October through February –
- Zinc, a mineral that helps prevent viral infections
  10 – 25 milligrams once or twice a day with food

- Vitamin C with bioflavonoids, boosts white blood cell immune system strength
  500 milligrams once or twice a day

At the *first sign* of a cold or flu –
Do the following FOR 4 DAYS consistently – symptoms may be gone by that time
- Zinc, a mineral that prevents a virus from attaching itself to a healthy human cell
  25 – 50 milligrams 3 times a day with food

- Vitamin C with bioflavonoids, a vitamin that boosts the immune system
  500 – 1000 milligrams 3 times a day

- Black Elderberry, helps reduce cough, chest congestion, and upper respiratory symptoms
  1 teaspoon of a liquid extract or syrup 3 times a day
    Can add this to a juice or water.

- Lomatium, a plant-based liquid valuable for reducing influenza and other viral infections
  5 *drops* of a liquid product, 3 times a day (a rash may appear, but will soon go away)
    Can add this to a juice or water, or combine with the black elderberry extract (above).

For product help for ordering: www.DSSorders.com/OHR Access code CY411
See "Resources Page' at the back of the book for product name suggestions.

Given the climate of the times, with rumors of devious terrorist tactics, and the recent announcement that the flu vaccines are going to be late and limited again, this year more than ever, we need to do all we can to be ready for fall and winter with a strong immune system. (Given the importance of this topic, and the amount of information I want to offer, look for two more parts on this subject to follow.)

As a naturopathic doctor, I know we have many ways to prevent disease, whether it is bacterial or viral of origin. Everything from prevention, to strong antiviral botanical medicine, to disease-fighting nutrients and diet, to hydrotherapy, to immune-boosting detoxification programs can be utilized to strengthen our immune systems. Each of these therapies offer assistance to staying healthy, helping to fend off colds and flu, and lending assistance in the effort to stay strong during times of physical and emotional times.

It is our immune system that defends us against disease-causing microorganisms and that supports the healing process. And it has been said that the process of aging is connected more to the immune system that that of the passing of time.

Weakening of the immune system results in greater susceptibility to virtually all illnesses. Some of the common signs of a depleted, or compromised, immune system are fatigue, frequent illness, allergic reactions, slow wound healing, skin eruptions, vaginal yeast infections, and chronic diarrhea.

Many factors contribute to a less than perfect immune system. A toxic environment and an unhealthy diet are on the top of the list. The more toxic load our system has to "throw off," the less capability it has to handle the normal day-to-day infectious encounters. That means that dirty hands, a sneeze in a crowded room, or a brisk chill on the neck can become more of a health threat than it normally is.

Other immune depressing contributors include chronic stress, smoking cigarettes, a change in the weather to a more humid climate, decreased hormone levels, lack of exercise, depressed state of mind, and consuming white refined and sugary foods. According to James F. Balch, MD, author of *Prescription for Nutritional Healing*, stress results in a sequence of biochemical events that ultimately suppresses the normal activity of white blood cells and places undue demands on the endocrine system, as well as depleting the body of needed nutrients. This is the greatest source of depletion for many people, and one that we especially need to protect ourselves against during these very trying days.

Hippocrates said, "Let your food be your medicine and your medicine be your food." So, before trying to supplement yourself back to health, look at a few simple health choices in your diet that will give your system a natural boost.

Foods with antiviral activity are very important, of course, since drug medicines have little to offer against viruses. As both an antiviral and an antibacterial, garlic is one of the strongest medicine foods on earth. It kills, on contact, all types of bacteria, making it a broad-spectrum antibiotic (known as "Russian Penicillin").

Garlic has also been shown to be powerful enough to destroy various viruses that cause upper respiratory infections and influenza. Keep garlic on hand and ready to eat raw at the first sign of illness. Other antiviral foods include apples, ginger, grapes, lemon juice, peaches, strawberries, sage, and those with glutathione (asparagus, avocado, oranges, and watermelon).

Foods that are rich in beta-carotene boost immune function. These are the orange and dark green pigmented ones such as (in order of most to least) dried apricots, cooked sweet potatoes, carrots, collard greens, kale, spinach, pumpkin, and cantaloupe. (Beta-carotene is not destroyed by cooking, according to USDA tests.) Most of the foods mentioned here have an abundance of vitamin C, too, another food component important in stimulating immunity. Others high on the vitamin C content list (in order of most to least) are guava, red sweet pepper, cantaloupe, sweet green pepper, papaya, grapefruit juice (if your medications allow it), tomatoes, and orange juice.

For the best immune system function avoid processed foods, sodas, coffee, and sugar. Sugar feeds cancer cells, plus yeast, bacteria, and parasites. A diet high in refined sugar does not feed you; it feeds disease. Sugar depletes the very white blood cells we need to fight disease, leaving us more vulnerable to disease.

It won't take much to stay well this fall. Specific food choices, support from natural therapeutics (that you will read about in the next article), and some common sense will go a long way in keeping our immune system up and running.

* * *

OUR BEST DEFENSE: A STRONG IMMUNE SYSTEM – 2

These days remind me of "preparing for The Millennium."

Fear of the unknown was pervasive and, in the end, many of us ended up with a garage full of powdered milk, canned goods, and generators we never used.

Today, it is gas masks that top the most-sought-after list, but the fear and uncertainty of whether we are "prepared" is still the same. Certainly, it is wise to error on the side of caution, especially when our transportation systems are being threatened. And whether it is hurricane-preparedness or any other threat to our safety, it may be smart to keep a few survival essentials on hand (www.fema.gov).

I say turn loose of the fear, and focus on our personal health and strength, knowing that undue stress will make our health worse, and tending to ourselves will help us gain more of the control we need to stay positive.

There may be something to be said, though, for preparedness. With the flu vaccines being late again this year, and more and more drug resistant bacteria on the rise, serious thought needs to be given to what else we can do to be ready for exposure to bacteria or virus.

Although unconventional throughout much of the medical community, recent research points to powerful botanical medicines with action now known to be antibacterial, antiviral, and antifungal. I suggest you either plant them in your yard or buy them now so you have quick access to them in the coming weeks.

Most of these names are unfamiliar to everyone except those closely involved in natural medicines. However, with the threat of limited medical resources looming in the future, it is a good idea to devote some time learning about them. Whereas, synthetic medicines usually have one active ingredient, a plant medicine is a multi-ingredient complex, making it actually hundreds on medicines in one. Of course, I like these consumed whole, raw, and fresh, or at least from a manufacturer who is either a laboratory or a research company.

The top 15 antibiotic plants are acacia, aloe, shiitake mushroom, echinacea, eucalyptus, garlic, ginger, goldenseal, grapefruit seed extract (GSE), pure wildflower honey, licorice (not the candy), sage, usnea, and wormwood. This list was derived from analyzing their length of use in folk medicine, beneficial outcomes in modern clinical practice, and results from modern scientific studies, including human studies. Recognize any? It would be wise to get familiar with them, have them, use them, and be healthy when others may not be.

Of this list my favorite natural antibiotics are raw garlic, grapefruit seed extract (GSE) and usnea (Old Man's Beard). GSE and garlic are two of the most powerful broad-spectrum antibiotics available for use, GSE surpassing the power of garlic by a considerable margin, as GSE used in small doses is quite effective. Clinical research on grapefruit seed extract shows antimicrobial effects against common bacteria such as: 86 strains of *E. coli*, *H. influenza*, *salmonella*, *M. tuberculosis*, 249 species of *staphylococcus*, 86 species of *streptococcus*, *candida*, *chlamydia*, *H. pylori*, and *influenza A2* virus. (Please note that this is grapefruit seed and pulp, not grape seed extract, the antioxidant.)

Usnea is strongly immune stimulating and possesses strong antibiotic properties, especially against gram-positive bacteria. Its usnic acid has shown activity more effective than penicillin against some bacterial strains, and found to completely inhibit the growth of organisms. Usnea has been traditionally used throughout the world for skin infections, abscesses, upper respiratory and lung infections, vaginal infections, and fungal infections, with no toxicity reported with oral therapeutic administration.

Those plant medicines that are particularly effective against viruses are lomatium, echinacea, garlic, grapefruit seed extract, and goldenseal. Others less well-known antivirals from plants include pau d'arco, shiitake mushroom, acemannan, and the sterols and sterolins from fruits and vegetables. Siberian ginseng is also helpful in improving resistance.

Although still considered a food, garlic deserves special attention. In World War I, garlic juice was applied to injuries. Again, in World War II, when antibiotics were not available to them, the Russians used garlic for battle wounds and thus it became known as Russian Penicillin. Garlic is best raw due to its potent sulfur (not sulfa) and allicin content, which is reduced when it is cooked or packaged for sale. It can be chopped or ground in juice or foods. The best way to eat raw garlic is to slice a sliver small enough to swallow, and then swallow without chewing it.

Besides the cancer-fighting sulfur content in garlic, it contains selenium, one of the best immune-boosting nutrients (more on nutrients and supplements in the next article). Garlic also has the ability to help the body detoxify heavy metals, especially mercury. Heavy metal toxicity is a serious burden to the immune system.

Virus, bacteria, and parasites pose constant challenges to the immune system. By their very nature, they are constantly changing, ever disguising themselves to avoid detection. Certainly the longer they are left to their own devices to more they multiply and growth in strength by their numbers. Our job is to keep them in check, low in numbers, with our complex disease-fighting system always on "high alert."

86

Begin to strengthen your immune system now. Start getting more rest, stay away from sugar, and begin to build your Emergency Health Kit today.

It is up to us, and only us, to be prepared.

Written and published October 14, 2001

* * *

Our Best Defense: A Strong Immune System – 3

Are you shopping for Halloween candy, or picking up the supplies you need to stock your medicine cabinet for emergency preparedness? My observation recently around town is strongly suggesting, "Shopping for candy."

Shocking as it may be, the threat of bio-terrorism is real; devoting a little thought now to preparation for the very remote chance that it may come here, may be important. If you have not listened to national news lately, or recently accessed Internet links regarding "preparedness", I am here to inform you that there is growing concern that perhaps we, as a country, may not be medically ready for such an attack.

Recently, Charles Simone, MD and immunologist, appeared on the Fox News. His message was 'How to Prepare Yourself for a Bio-terrorist Attack'. These were simple, common sense ways we should know and already be doing. Second on his list, just after "be alert," was to "boost your immune system." His description matches mine in ways to naturally prepare your health against a microorganism that could deplete our well-being. And whether the threat of anthrax, smallpox, plague, botulism, E. boli, or tularemia is as threatening as some have advised that it is (and as history has shown them to be), we know that cold and flu season is none-the-less just around the corner, both of harmful bacterial and virus in origin.

Dr. Simone said that even though the drugs, cipro and doxycycline, are the drugs of choice to treat anthrax, he and others agree that neither may be available to a large population of people should a harmful fate fall upon great numbers.

What action is left? Get your shopping done now, but put your money in immune-supporting nutrients, not the sugar that depletes our health. Buy the best you can afford, leaving cheap over-the-counter supplements alone this time. Remember, you get what you pay for.

While these may be part, but not all, of the natural medicine treatment plan designed to stave off the stronger strains, make sure you have at least these on hand: zinc, vitamin C, selenium, echinacea, goldenseal, and lots of raw garlic.

When you suspect an illness is approaching, whether it is the cold or flu, or another unknown disease, these are to be taken at high dosages for a short time for treatment, and at lower doses for prevention. Do not try to dose yourself at treatment doses without the advice of a licensed doctor, as the wrong combination or dosages may interact with present medications or each other, or you may all short of an effective dosage. (Treatments for the more life-threatening bacteria and viruses will require the more complex formula.)

If you or your family members are not already in touch with a naturopathic doctor, contact the American Association of Naturopathic Physicians at 866-538-2267 (www.naturopathic.org) for one in their area. This group is trained in detoxification of harmful agents, lymphatic massage for boosting immune function, hydrotherapy for internal cleansing and nourishing, and medical nutrition for therapeutically treating complex illnesses. Before Sept. 11, doctors of naturopathic medicine were busy formulating natural hormone replacement for women, helping patients lower their cholesterol without drugs, and treating complex conditions.

Recently, however, they have banded together as a strong network of practitioners, burning the midnight oil, to develop effective non-drug methods and therapies to counter the deadly effects from disease-causing biological organisms, diseases thought in conventional medical circles today as being "non-curable." Some skeptics may remind us that they are "not FDA approved," and that is correct, as these are not synthetic drugs, but medicines of a natural resource, not falling under the jurisdiction of the FDA.

Those who were saved from the deadly plague many years ago having been treated with botanicals, and those who were HIV positive and still living healthy lives today from treatment with immune-system supportive Chinese bitter melon (*momordica charanchia*), probably did not care if these natural medicines were FDA approved or not.

These are times in which we are all scrambling for answers. It is a time when we must look "outside the box" and begin to entertain the prospects of alternative ways to protect our health. Given the rise in antibiotic-resistance diseases, it is time to give serious thought to the healing power of nature.

It has been said that God gave us all the medicines we need, already surrounding us in nature. Perhaps now is the time, more than ever, to recognize them.

Written and published on October 21, 2001

* * *

FOOD

FORTIFY YOUR CEREAL SNACKS - QUICKLY AND EASILY

Boxed-suppers are not what they used to be. Today, many of us are eating our supper out of store-bought cereal boxes, due to time constraints on shopping and cooking. Despite the list of vitamins and minerals proudly displayed on the carton side column, surely you must know that something is missing.

If you have not gotten into box reading, now is the time to start. I almost fainted flat on the ground from shock last week when I saw the simple basic snack, the Vanilla Wafer, now being offered in bright, fun-filled, colors. Reading its long list of ingredients revealed many of them to be not only sugars, bad enough, but also including many toxic dyes considered to be cancer-causing by many. One more boxed-snack now questionable in its health benefits.

An interesting combination in boxed-cereals these days is the zero-to-small amounts of vitamin C and zinc (read for yourself), and the large amounts of sugars and wheat (gluten). This recipe is not only a poor combination if we intend to keep our immune system strong, since we need both these vitamins for this function, but the sugar brings our energy and immune system down while many people have food sensitivities to wheat.

Often with this nutrient-deficient combination we could find ourselves getting sick easier, and being plagued by unexplained allergy symptoms on top of that from all the mucous-forming wheat.

I cannot advise you whether or not to base your evening meal on a bowl of cereal (or to munch on a red or blue snack wafer), because obviously boxed foods leave a lot to be desired as a safe or complete meal choice. But I can tell you how to boost its nutritional content, helping you to milk your cereal for all its worth as a snack choice.

You will need a coffee grinder, and a Tupperware-type plastic sealed container or glass jar to make this natural food additive. Ingredients you will need are: oats, milk thistle seeds, flax seeds, sunflower seeds, lecithin, and maybe some cinnamon or nutmeg.

Grind the seeds in the grinder and put all ingredients in the container, stir it up, seal it tightly and refrigerate. When hit by a desire for a quick cereal snack, sprinkle a tablespoon of this nutrient-rich mix on top of your cereal to boost its vitamin, mineral, and fiber content.

The milk thistle is a great liver detoxifying herb. The oils from the flaxseeds and sunflower seeds are sources of essential fatty acid oils used for arthritis, to prevent heart attacks by lowering cholesterol, and to relieve constipation. Lecithin granules help to reduce fatty accumulation in liver, is used for treating dementia, and also to reduce high cholesterol. Cinnamon is a digestive stimulant, used to reduce gas (also nutmeg), lower high blood glucose, and to help stop diarrhea. Oat bran, of course, is a high-fiber food and beneficial for cholesterol levels by decreasing cholesterol absorption, and important for reducing the risk of colon cancer. Do not worry about cooking the oats; it is chewy and delicious just like it comes out of its box.

If you do not have a grinder, a similar recipe can be concocted for cereal lovers by chopping or using of a mortar and pestle and, as above, can be prepared ahead of time, kept in the refrigerator, and added to cereals any time of day for that extra nutrient boost.

Combine raisins or other dried fruits, wheat germ, oats, bran, sunflower seeds, almonds, pumpkin seeds, walnuts, and/or lecithin into the a big sealable container. (Use raw and unsalted seeds for your best health.) The consistency should be similar to a dry, high fiber, homemade granola mix without all the sticky sugar or syrup. And speaking of sugar, make sure you top your cereal with stevia if you require a sweetener, not sugar, aspartame, saccharin, or sucralose/Splenda®.

If you are lactose intolerant pick the proper milk source that is best for you, such as almond milk. You may get to liking this natural cereal you have just made so much that you might want to use it without the basic store-bought boxed cereals. It is a good idea, though, to increase your water intake, given the increased fiber you will be consuming.

If you have a hard time finding these ingredients, do your best to design your own recipe based on your available resources. Your base cereal, though, like Grape-Nuts or Raisin Bran, should be sugar free and high in fiber. You can also add a couple of tablespoons of this high-fiber mix to a meat loaf, a casserole, or in other vitamin-depleted boxed-snacks, depending on what spices you include in your recipe.

Making this quick 'Mighty-Mix' recipe of chopped nuts or seeds, raisins, and rolled oats or bran will stay refrigerator-fresh for a long time, will make your cereal snack more satisfying and nutritious, and keep your heart, liver, and colon a whole lot happier.

* * *

Organic Food Issue: Getting to the Root of It

What's in a name these days? More importantly, what's in a food? There seems to be a lot of confusion over what is "organic" and what is not. As expensive as it commonly is to purchase organic from the grocery stores, can we trust the quality of our purchases from the roadside vendors offering what they label as organically grown goodies to save money, and feel certain they are truly organic? The answer is that it depends on what standard one uses.

The definition of "organic" is: foods that are grown without the use of synthetic chemicals, such as pesticides, herbicides, and hormones. However, according to the United States Department of Agriculture, they not only must be grown without the topical use of these harmful chemicals, but grown in pesticide-free soil as well.

To be "certified organic," assuring the toxin-free process actually is guaranteed, the USDA must give their seal of approval to the soil in which the crops are grown, requiring it to be pesticide-free for three years, the time they feel it takes pesticides to leach out from the soil.

Unfortunately, this leaves out most roadside produce stands, those good-intentioned folks who strive for better living without chemistry. While their hearts are in the right place, they probably fall short of the strict standards required for public sale by the USDA.

I've been told that the sale of organic foods is "down" in some stores, given the higher prices due to spoilage on those unprotected and unpreserved portions of the crops. Yet, many people continue to ask for it, searching for the pesticide-free food resources that they insist be represented and available to them.

How do you tell the certified organics just by looking? Usually a typical unwrapped produce item will be displayed with a four-digit number on its sticker. Certified organics are marked, however, with a 5-digit number, beginning with "9." They come directly from the farms labeled this way. You can also check with the produce manager. They should be able to show you the box in which the foods arrived, which should bear the certification label declaring its organic origin "in accordance with the California Organic Food Act of 1990." Some may also come marked with a similar certification from Washington State, another location of strict organic food farms.

Each farm then must be licensed and regularly inspected by the USDA so that strict standards are maintained. Food stores, too, are subject to spot checks by government representatives, and anyone selling produce advertised as "organic" which is not, under the guidelines of the USDA, is subject to harsh fines.

Choosing organic foods is a huge health improvement step despite the price. We applaud growers who decline the use of pesticides and other toxic chemicals as part of their growing process. Nevertheless, we especially thank the USDA for requiring that pesticides be free from the soil as well.

Wouldn't it be nice if the soils were not only pesticide-free, but also nutrient-rich? However, that's a concern sprouting up of another subject, entirely.

* * *

THE "POWER" IN PROTEIN POWDERS

Why all the interest in protein powders these days? We see canisters of them on the shelves of health food stores, in gyms, and in some doctors' offices. Contents describing everything from "whey" to "soy" to "amino acids" are seen. What does it all mean and why is it important to learn about them?

Amino acids are the building blocks (or 'pieces') upon which our dietary protein is made. It is the smaller amino acids our body needs and can use, not necessarily the 'whole' protein provided in the form of our dietary beef and chicken.

Of the 28 amino acids, some are made in the body by a functioning liver and the others must be obtained from the diet.

Most amino acids support muscle health as well as ligaments, tendons, organs, glands, nails, hair, and bones. Additionally, they are important for optimal detoxification of toxins held in the body. The huge science of amino acid proteins can be chewed down to a smaller bite by saying that we need all of the amino acids to function and many of us just aren't getting them.

These days our dietary protein comes from many sources, much of it from animals that may have been raised on steroids or treated with antibiotics, or both; it's a source of protein that often comes with an automatic side of gristle, fat, and bone. Our protein-rich eggs may also come from a source of stressed or poorly nourished hens.

It is no wonder that many people opt not to partake of animal protein foods these days; many choose to stick with the vegetables they know and love. Unfortunately, complete protein is not found in plants, and therefore we need an auxiliary source of protein to maintain muscle strength and energy. With the exception of soybeans, vegetable proteins are usually lacking in one or two essential amino acids. A mixture of vegetable proteins from different sources, however, each with a relative, but different deficit in essential amino acids, can make for a more wholesome "complete" or ideal mixture.

Without the "essential amino acids", those proteins that our body does not naturally produce, many ill-health symptoms may arise. A deficiency in methionine, for example, has been linked with chemical allergies as this amino acid helps to detoxify harmful agents from the body; a lack of histidine could result in a lower white or red blood cell count, as its job is to help increase and build both; and a low level of tryptophan may alter brain serotonin levels, a neurotransmitter that assists in normal sleep and helps stabilize mood and combat depression.

The combination of what is called the "branched chain amino acids" (BCAA) is particularly important for those who exercise or have fibromyalgia. Both groups need muscle-healing nutrients. These three amino acids - isoleucine, leucine, and valine - are primary building blocks of muscle tissue and are used by the muscles during exercise to supply energy. In addition, as all three are "essential" (meaning that it is *essential* we add them to our diet), if we do not restock our bodies of these we could experience fatigue, muscle pain, or tissue deterioration. Muscle size and strength can also diminish.

A good source of BCAA is found in whey protein, a high quality protein resource important in maintaining muscle structure, improving immune function, repairing muscle, and promoting muscle growth. Remember, it is these three amino acids that are used most frequently by the muscles as an energy source, so their replacement through the diet is "essential." As a dairy protein, however, whey protein (and another milk protein, casein) could cause mild gastrointestinal symptoms in dairy-sensitive individuals.

Amino acids are assisted in forming their full protein molecules in the body with the help of vitamin C and vitamin B6. The active form of vitamin B6, pyridoxyl-5-phosphate, is preferred.

Some popular supplements are basically just single amino acids. '5-HTP' is actually a form of the essential amino acid, tryptophan; and 'SAMe' is methionine by another name. Both these popular supplements are promoted as therapies to relieve depression and pain and to help induce sleep.

It makes sense to build our much-needed hormones and neurotransmitters from dietary protein sources. For example, tryptophan is a building block of serotonin (the good mood neurotransmitter) and melatonin (the sleep hormone). Found in turkey meat, tryptophan is sleep promoting and is one of the reasons we are often sleepy after a Thanksgiving meal. A do-at-home urine test to determine the level of neurotransmitters in your system is available. Once a NEI SuperSystem-trained professional (a NeuroScience Inc. certification) reviews the results, a 'targeted amino-acid' program can be designed to help rebuild those deficient neurotransmitters.

Limited public 'press' has been given to amino acids and their importance for mental and physical health. Consequently, many overlook the role they play in the total health of our bodies. However, it is from these basic building blocks of protein nutrients that the miracle of faster tissue repair, increased energy levels, pain relief, and physical endurance can often be attained.

* * *

THE GREATNESS OF GRAPEFRUIT

In 1978, the World Health Organization (WHO) passed a resolution stating their intent that all people in the world should have adequate health care by the year 2000. This meant they claimed that therapy sources other than western or conventional pharmaceutical medicine would have to be accessed and utilized for this goal to be met. The report concluded with the recommendation that the values and benefits of centuries-old herbal medicine be pursued through research in order to meet the emerging health needs of the exploding world population.

The historic research resulting from this resolution adopted by WHO discovered and revisited the fact that global medicines of our forefathers included many plants that possess strong antibacterial qualities. In many instances they are equal to, and may even surpass, the power of today's conventional antibiotics.

One of these is grapefruit seed and pulp, or 'grapefruit seed extract', a powerful broad-spectrum (kills many strains) natural antibiotic. (This is not to be confused with grape seed extract.) GSE, as it is sometimes called, is often marketed under the name, Citricidal®. According to their published research, it is active against yeasts, fungus, bacteria, viruses, worms, and parasites.

Generally, GSE is professionally manufactured from the seed and pulp (inside the peel) of the grapefruit. The exact process is a closely kept secret, but it is not unreasonable to assume that a simple home extractor procedure should work as well, using the seeds and pulp. Note that its bitter taste can best be disguised in an equally citric fruit juice, such as orange, grapefruit, lemonade, and limeade. Capsules containing GSE are used successfully for internal conditions without any aftertaste.

Though it has proved impossible to discover the process used to commercially make Citricidal®, there is significant evidence that the grapefruit plant and all the citrus family possess potent antibacterial activity, thus the custom of including a slice of lemon served atop a glass of water when it is dispensed as tap water.

Usually Citricidal® Liquid Extract is formulated with 60% GSE and 40% glycerin, a sweetening and soothing agent often used in medicines. This smooth emollient ingredient makes it easier for the mucous membranes to tolerate its powerful antibiotic action. It is popularly and effectively used as a nasal spray to fight sinus infections, and has no uncomfortable side effects that some pharmaceuticals can cause.

Grapefruit seed extract is used by naturopathic physicians, and more recently some conventional medical doctors to kill strep, staph, salmonella, E. coli, herpes, influenza, candida, H. pylori, and other microbes that cause diarrhea, stomach ulcers, depressed immune function, allergies, candida, and infections. It is also in widespread use as a drinking water treatment and as a disinfectant for toothbrushes, meats, fish, poultry, fruits, vegetables, cutting boards and as an extremely effective additive to laundry and dish soap as it ensures adequate disinfection of clothing, linens, and eating utensils.

Citricidal® provides killing action of microbes without the toxicity inherent in harmful chemicals. In studies comparing its disinfectant power against chlorine and iodine, grapefruit seed extract was dramatically more effective in inhibiting growth of the organisms mentioned above than other agents tested.

As a natural alternative to pharmaceutical antibiotics, grapefruit seed extract is non-toxic and non-corrosive making it safe for infants and elderly, as well as those with compromised health. Besides being as effective as a nasal spray, GSE is used in toothpastes, dental rinses, eardrops, shampoo, and as facial cleaners, vaginal douches, and for nail treatment.

Grapefruit seed extract is not to be used undiluted due to its powerful effect at full strength. Always make sure that your purchase resource understands its potential and its potency and is able to answer your questions regarding the proper proportion of dilution before you begin treatment.

Grapefruit seed extract is the best-kept secret in modern medicine. With research supporting its benefits, why is it so unknown in the United States and under-used by our doctors as a powerful antibiotic and treatment resource? Who knows? Perhaps the World Health Organization can answer that.

* * *

SPICES: THE FORGOTTEN MEDICINES OF LIFE

Hippocrates, the Father of Medicine and author of our medical Hippocratic Oath, said, "Let your food be your medicine, and your medicine be your food." This, too, is part of the naturopathic physician's oath and philosophy for health repair without medications.

In this fast-paced world of supplement-selling and pill-pushing, it is easy to forget the value of what lies right before us: the simple medicines found in spices.

Spices are rich in phytonutrients. Phytonutrients are compounds in food plants that have anti-oxidant, anti-inflammatory, anti-cancer, anti-toxin, and many other health-promoting properties. Spices can prevent diseases. Extensive medical research has found that nutrients in ginger, turmeric, rosemary, fenugreek, oregano, cloves and many other spices can help to prevent heart disease, Alzheimer's, cancer, diabetes and other degenerative diseases.

Spices have the highest antioxidant activity of all foods and provide the variety of antioxidants needed to protect athletes and other highly active people from oxidative stress and accelerated aging.

Back in Biblical times, spices were traded as a monetary commodity – on par with gold and silver. Spices are often still used in rituals, as they are highly valued for their medicinal properties.

Unfortunately, throughout the years, the value of spices has changed from 'health promoting' to 'food seasoning'. We think of our spices as additives to food, and have forgotten the medicinal value of spices. Today, they have been shuffled to the back of our cabinets, letting them age until we finally throw them away as too old to use.

Depending on what the medical goal is, I choose from a variety of fresh ground spices. I select from my fresh resource of 'bulk, organic' spices at a quality health food store, not off the shelf at a big box or discount grocery store.

Here are some my favorite medicinal spices and their uses.

Turmeric is in the ginger family of plants and is sometimes called, yellow ginger. Turmeric (curcumin) has anti-inflammatory properties, is healthy to the liver and gallbladder, and is cancer preventative.

An increasing body of scientific research is showing turmeric to be one of the most valuable medicinal spices with potent preventive and, in some cases, therapeutic effects against a variety of serious chronic diseases such as cancer and Alzheimer's disease. When measured against other phytonutrients, or natural plant chemicals, that protect against cancer, turmeric exhibits at least a ten times greater cancer protective potency than its closest rival.

Ginger, another favorite, helps prevent cardiovascular disease in several ways. It has been shown to lower dangerously high cholesterol and triglyceride levels, while raising the levels of beneficial HDL. And like turmeric, ginger has anti-cancer benefits and can reduce pain. Its hot taste can increase the metabolic rate (metabolism), thus helping in weight loss and helps prevent diabetes by supporting our natural glucose-lowering processes.

Together with turmeric, ginger has protection against dementia and Alzheimer's and has been said to reverse the amyloid plaque in the brain associated with memory loss.

One of the active compounds in another of my favorites, rosemary, is carnosic acid. Unlike many other herbs and spices, the oils of rosemary can cross the blood-brain-barrier to help dilate blood vessels in the brain. By doing this, rosemary supports two of the major arteries carrying blood to the brain. Increased blood flood in the brain can increase oxygen and nutrients being delivered throughout the brain. This is just one reason rosemary is associated with "remembrance." A strong and effective antioxidant, we will sometimes find rosemary added to supplements, such as fish oil, to prevent them from turning old or rancid. It works the same way in our bodies, as the antioxidant that it is.

Cilantro is both an herb and a spice. A member of the carrot family, the leaves are classified as an herb, its seeds are called coriander. I like to use the leaves, as it is helpful in detoxification of heavy metals from the body, such as mercury and lead. Cilantro is sold as a fresh herb by-the-bunch in the produce section of most markets. It is also easy to grow, however, and less expensive this way.

A therapeutic blend of fresh spices might replace many of your old store-bought supplements, if chosen properly. A customized blend should, at the very least, be part of every health program.

* * *

WEIGHT MANAGEMENT

How to be Well on Your Weigh – 1

Since we know that 'wherever our mind goes our body will follow', it is essential that our mind lead the way to proper weight management.

Our weight loss program begins with understanding first why it is we want to lose weight, and to decide if it is an important enough reason to devote time to making it into a project. Why a project? Because unless we do, it will slide into our "never gets done" list. It has to become a priority, an intent…a project for which we make time and devote some effort.

First, get straight with what is driving this desire to lose weight. Did someone suggest it? A doctor, friend, or spouse? Do you consider the extra pounds to be a health hazard? Do you have clothes in our closet that don't fit? Or, maybe all of the above?

There is a very real concept called 'emotional weight', whereby we add those extra pounds as we unconsciously nibble ourselves into obesity in order to fill an emotional hole created by the loss of a loved one, nervousness, stress, or boredom. This kind of eating habit is akin to smoking, a bad habit just needing to be broken. Make your unconscious habit conscious (and thus, easier to break) and decide to repair your emotional damage in healthful ways.

For some people, understanding the 'why' is all it takes. No use making a bad situation even worse from habitual, unintentional eating. Deciding to lose weight for someone else is not a strong enough reason to start a program. Without your own personal involvement, commitment, and planning, nothing changes.

Once you have determined your motivation for losing weight, and have made the decision for long-term dedication to a program of simple changes, you are off and running…or walking. Keep in mind that the number on the scale should not be the gauge of your success. Some simple, yet continual, changes will lead you to both a smaller number on the scale, and a smaller size. If you are looking for the quick weight loss program, sorry, this is not it. It is, however, the program that is designed for permanent health benefits.

Our simple program will have three basic parts: eliminate sugar and sugary foods, add more activity to slightly increase your normal heart rate, and stay focused and committed. It is a simple, yet effective method. (Update: See the Amazon book, *Sleep More, Weigh Less'* by T. Shepherd)

Let's deal with the last one first, as this is probably the most important. Until we make up our mind that many of the foods that we have loved may not love us, our efforts here will fail. When we begin to add up the sugar we consume on a daily basis, as you will learn to do, or realize how we constantly are munching on junk food through the day and night, we soon realize that a change is essential.

Until we realize that we must find time through the day to include some activity, we will continue to pack on the pounds. Until we are ready to be healthy, we will continue to need to make changes. So, understand now, that this is not only weight management, but also optimal health training, and that this is not a temporary change, but a change for life.

Consider finding a friend, doctor, email pen pal, or personal trainer to support you in your changes, if necessary. By working as a team or in partnership, it will be easier to make the right decisions, stay focused, and will be more fun.

Begin now by looking through your house, office, and car for foods that are high in sugar, or other simple carbohydrates, and throw them out. These foods are candies, doughnuts, soft drinks, crackers, pastries, cookies, cakes, ice cream, and sugary breakfast cereals. Even with kids in the house, reduce these foods as much as possible to avoid being tempted, and to keep the kids from the perils of obesity, as well.

Keep in mind that our program will involve avoidance of sugar through the week with more leniencies on the weekends. By allowing for a 5 day detox from sugar, we reduce our sugar cravings, become slimmer, protect our teeth from decay, have more energy, less digestive problems, and less allergies just to name a few. Start reducing your sugar intake *now*.

Remember that where the mind goes, the body will follow. It is just that simple. When you get your mind set for success, visualizing your goal, plan for foods that will nourish your weight loss, not hinder it, gather a support system, and begin to create time for exercise, you are well on your weigh.

* * *

He who has begun has half done.
Dare to be wise; begin!

HORACE

106

How to Be Well on Your Weigh – 2

In the last chapter, we discussed the importance of being mindfully ready to begin a weight loss program, to be thought of as a gradual change for the complete benefit of all body system. As we said, one key change is to drastically reduce your sugar intake, as sugar lends itself to fat storage if not used as energy, or if eaten with a fat resource food (as suggested in food-combining guidelines).

Start counting the sugar grams on the packages of the foods you consume, noticing the portion serving size. For more rapid weight loss, keep the sugar grams to less than 30 a day through the week. Notice the high sugar content especially in the soft drinks, breakfast cereals, and juices. Keep your sugar consumption to morning meals when your activity is ahead of you; do not sit at your desk or in front of the TV set or computer mindlessly munching on cookies, candy, or drinking pop. Mindless munching, remember, is a habit to break. Just stop doing it.

Remember that many foods turn into sugar once the digestion process begins. These are foods which are said to be high on the "glycemic index of carbohydrate foods." These foods stimulate insulin release, which creates a storage process of the foods contained within that meal. Consequently, when we eat a high glycemic food (sugar, white flour, baked potato, white or instant rice, corn, beer, crackers) in combination with a fatty food or ingredient, our bodies tend to store both as fat.

These combinations include: steak (with marbled fat) and potatoes, macaroni and cheese, most sandwiches that contain a fat, meat, or cheese source, hamburgers, cheese and crackers, beer and potato chips, baked potatoes with butter and sour cream, French-fries, tortilla chips, cakes, cookies, pies, and sugary cereals with whole milk, just to name a few common weight-gaining fat/carbohydrate combinations.

Food-combining is a fairly unknown concept, but well documented throughout many resources as advanced biochemistry. A complete article should be devoted to this subject, but for weight loss purposes, do not combine a high fat resource with a simple carbohydrate or starchy food in the same meal. The result will be sluggish metabolism, plus a tendency to store both the fat and the carbohydrate in the fat cells. A steak or another fatty food resource like avocados, cheese, or dairy, eaten with a vegetable or salad (without bread or crackers) is less harmful on weight management than most people would think when we eliminate the crackers and bread in the same meal. Once the pancreas has to activate its insulin from a food that creates sugar in the system, we had better have all fatty foods or ingredients out of our stomach to avoid weight gain.

Although nature will takes its due weight loss course with the simple diet and exercise modifications, there are supplements (called "anti-fat nutrients") that will indeed shorten the weight loss time. First, let me say that I do not like ephedra, ephedrine, and Ma Huang in a weight loss program. There are too many medical complications and adverse reactions from both and there are better nutrients with no harmful effects.

I particularly like the amino acid L-carnitine, which is also used therapeutically to reduce cholesterol, triglycerides, and LDLs, and to increase HDL (good cholesterol) in the blood. This is the nutrient that helps to move fat out of the tissues and into the part of the cell that produces the energy molecule. What a great combination: less body fat, more energy, and better heart health! It does take the proper supportive nutrients to activate this process, so consult a doctor trained in nutritional medicine to identity the proper dosages of each. Sometimes people not able to lose weight are actually deficient of this protein and with its addition, find their program to be successful.

As with L-carnitine, coenzyme Q10 and pantethine (vitamin B-5) may also prove to be of benefit to those who are overweight because they also are essential in the proper transport and breakdown of fat into energy. Nutrients that support thyroid function are also good. These are kelp, bladderwrack, selenium, and L-tyrosine (the natural building block of the thyroid hormone). Diuretics can be supportive as well, such as lemon, apple cider vinegar, and grapefruit, but bear in mind that cells will usually rehydrate once the diet changes again.

Sugar cravings are often reduced with the help of the mineral, chromium, at proper dosages, and another amino acid protein called L-glutamine. Remember, that the elimination of sugar is still the best way to change this craving.

An important natural agent that may help to prevent the production of fat and suppress appetite is call *Garcinia cambogia*. Although studies support fat production inhibition in animals, it has not yet been proven in human studies. It only inhibits the conversion of carbohydrates into fat; therefore, it will have little effect on dietary fat.

In the next article, we will move into our next step of weight management, exercise. Take this opportunity to find your comfortable, yet arch-supportive, pair of shoes and start to find and organize your workout clothes. Keep it simple, basic, and easy since the dress code for going to the gym, or walking in the neighborhood, is not the same as going to the theater.

If you are with us at this point, and well on your weigh, congratulations. Hang in there and keep up the good work! Rome was not built in a day, nor does weight become "lost" overnight.

* * *

Thus far, our weight management has been simple: Make up your mind to make the changes you've needed to make for your overall health, eliminate sugar from your diet, as well as most simple carbohydrates (crackers, cakes, cookies, and other sugary foods) and reduce other carbs that are high on the glycemic index such as white potatoes, instant rice, and white bread, especially while eating a food that has fat in it, such as described in the principles of food-combining.

The key to this program is understanding that carbohydrates stimulate insulin production. Insulin lowers blood sugar (a good thing), but it also converts glucose and protein into fat, and converts dietary fat to storage (a bad thing). Raising insulin by eating a simple carbohydrate, also increases the body's production of cholesterol, makes the kidneys retain excess fluid leading to high blood pressure, and basically shifts metabolism into a storage mode.

Though he does not always make it clear, this is the same biochemical principle behind Dr. Atkins' controversial high protein, high fat diet: When the carbohydrates are not present in the diet to raise blood sugar and ignite insulin production, our bodies release fat from fat cells and makes it available for energy, utilizes dietary fats for energy, helps release excess fluid from the kidney, shifting metabolism into a "burning" mode. The bottom line on all of this is that high glycemic index carbohydrates need to be limited during a weight loss program so that the production of insulin, the fat storing hormone, is not over-stimulated.

Our next important ingredient of this weight management program is, of course, movement. We have become a culture of moving from the bed to the computer, to the car, to the office, back home to the TV, back to bed. It has become an effort to move, and we are now paying the price for a sedentary existence. Muscles lose strength at a rate of about 12 to 14 percent per decade after age 50, it has been reported.

Aside from the benefits of weight loss, another important reason we exercise is to maintain the health of the cardiovascular and pulmonary system, those systems supplying the most essential nutrient of all to the cells of the body: oxygen.

In weight control, regular exercise will speed up the body's metabolic rate. It also stimulates the release of endorphins, the natural painkillers, from the brain. The most helpful type of exercise is aerobic. This is the type that increases the heart rate and makes you breathe harder. There are specific guidelines to follow to assure that your exercise is program is right for you, so check with your doctor before beginning this part. You should get a complete physical within one year before starting an exercise program.

Aerobic exercise includes walking, jogging, running, hiking, swimming, bicycling, rowing, dancing, tennis, and others. They are aerobic because they can be done continuously and steadily with no interruption for at least twelve minutes at a time and they are vigorous enough to assure that your heart will beat at the "training heart rate" for the entire twelve minutes.

First, do a slow version of the exercise you have chosen for three to five minutes to warm up, and then three to five minutes more to cool down after exercising. Second, gently stretch the muscles you are using both before and after exercising. Third, exercise a minimum of three to four times every week, preferably not on consecutive days.

When dieting, up to forty percent of weight loss is lean muscle mass. While losing weight you can protect muscle tissue with strength training and the amino acids we have already discussed in the earlier chapter on protein. An effective strength-training program must include several repetitions at a resistance that will "overload" the muscle, therefore building strength as you work out. Strength training has been proven to be a solution to permanent body fat reduction. It is also the most effective exercise format for maintaining bone density.

Exercise should be fun, not painful or dreaded. Build up your endurance safely, slowly, and progressively. It is crucial for building and maintaining health. Make it a part of this program, but make it a regular part of your life. The investment of time and energy into exercise will pay off in a better quality of life.

Do not panic with your weight, making you desperate to quickly see the scale reflect a lower number. Begin to make the changes and by doing so, change will come. If you are restricting your sugar and high glycemic carbohydrate foods, incorporating more movement in your routine, and are committed to a course of improved health and a slimmer you, congratulations. You are part of an elite group who are well on their weigh to optimal health.

* * *

101 REASONS TO EXERCISE

In a perfect world, doctors would meet their patients at the gym. After they had exercised, the docs would thank their patient, the patient would thank their doctor, and there would be no charge for medical counseling, no charge required for expensive medication, and no money paid out for supplements because there would be no need for any of these.

Research shows that regular exercise lowers the risk for many diseases, supporting virtually every system in the body to improve overall health and well-being. Why pay out hundreds or thousands of dollars for "repair," if our body does not have to break? Most people answer, "No time to exercise." To what, I ask, can be of more importance to devote your time than to your health?

An interesting and informative sign hangs above the drinking fountain at a local fitness center: 101 Reasons to Exercise, it says. It describes the statistic that fewer than 40% of Americans exercise enough to experience significant health benefits. I was impressed by the fact that the philosophy there is focused not just on weight loss and increasing muscle mass, but also on the total health gain attained through exercise. Hats off to this facility for supporting this philosophy and for helping to spread the word.

Here are some of the important, and little known, health reasons amongst those 101 listed there. These directly correlate to the physical complaints I hear repeatedly, that are costly to fix, if not through exercise:

Exercise helps reduce stress, improving the quality of sleep, and enhancing sexual performance and satisfaction. It increases the density and strength of bones, retarding bone loss, and slows the rate of joint degeneration in people prone to osteoporosis. (Bones respond to the stress of exercise by laying down more bone mineral deposits.)

Exercise decreases circulating triglycerides (fats in your blood), helping to eliminate the risk of heart disease, and making the heart a more efficient pump. Exercise decreases the risk of breast cancer and reduces the symptoms of menopause.

For diabetics, exercise increases tissue responsiveness to the action of insulin for better control of their diabetes. It protects against "creeping obesity" and decreases appetite. Those affected by depression should find improved self-esteem, better mental alertness, less anxiety, and more energy.

Muscles lose strength at a rate of about 12 to 14 percent per decade after age 50, reported in the *IDEA Health and Fitness Source Journal*. The losses in strength are probably due to shrinkage in muscle size. Again, however, strength training can make big changes. Two months of weight training can reverse as much as two decades of muscle shrinkage and strength loss, the article says.

By investing in exercise, instead of continually spending our hard-earned money on medications, we receive daily dividends and constant healthy paybacks, eventually getting on top of the health issue for good. Through medication without exercise, there may never be a correction, just medicating.

If those sedentary Americans would begin to exercise, it has been estimated that the savings on health costs would be about $80 billion dollars a year, by improving overall quality of life, as each inactive American spends about $330 more a year on health expenses than does the active American.

Next time your doctor calls you for a follow up appointment, see if he or she will meet you at the gym to do a workout. Having your best health at heart, they will have helped every system in your body, and helped themselves as well.

And in a real or imagined world of healthcare, what could be better than that?

* * *

SUPPLEMENTS & MEDICATIONS

SUPPLEMENT PLANNING: A PILL OF A PROJECT

So many supplements, so much confusion…what is one to do when it comes to planning a personal program for oneself?

If you are one who attended one of my classes, *"Supplements: The Good, the Bad, and the Toxic,"* you already have a basic understanding of where to proceed. If not, here is a quick outline that may help you.

Deciding on what supplements suit you require completing a little "homework," but the results are worth it. You will want to write down each section of information you will be asked to acquire in order to see the grand picture.

Begin by defining your health goals, that is, what you are trying to achieve through supplementation. Then make a list of the foods that you know may have been replacing the nutrient-rich foods you may have been needing. These are foods you will want to replace in order to get nutrients from food sources so as to reduce the need for supplementation.

Next, list those conditions in your family history that may contribute to your genetic picture. Even though you may not have seen any of these appear in your own health, it is important to support these "systems" so that problems seen in other family members do not begin to show up in you. Try to list not only mother and father, but siblings and grandparents as well as some conditions may skip a generation. You now need to add this family medical history information to your list of goals (heart health? bone health? cancer or stroke prevention?).

Our next step may be foreign to some of you if you have not worked with me in the past. It involves getting a copy of your past and current lab work copies from your doctor. You may have to go by their office and ask for them in person, or call the records department and request they send them to you. I would suggest you ask for lab work for the past two years. Most doctors are accustomed to this request by now and may charge you nothing, or at the very least, the cost of the copies.

Now, create your own file or three-ring-binder, label it "My Health," and put these reports in it. You should also always request copies of any radiology (x-rays, MRI, or CT scans) that were done when they are completed, but it is the blood work that will be most useful for designing your supplement program. Keep in mind that a normal value on a report may appear to be good, but it is when you compare it to a previous report you are able to determine if that particular lab value has gotten better or worse. It is then that you will really be able to determine what pattern of health is developing.

Now comes an even more remote concept, but still important in determining the overall nutrient need you may have. A new science is developing – that of nutrients being depleted from common medications. If you are on a number of drugs, my suggestion would be to do some research by getting the book, "Drug-Induced Nutrient Depletion Handbook." This is a 485-page reference that describes what vitamins or minerals may be removed from your body by taking drugs and is written by group of registered pharmacists. Each listing has a research reference to support its importance. (If the book is not available, do your own research on 'nutrients depleted by medications.')

One such notation says that estrogens deplete vitamin B6, important for good mood elevation, and magnesium, important for heart health and pain relief. Another page describes coenzyme Q10 as being depleted from the statin drugs, such as Lipitor®. Coenzyme Q10, the book says, is one of the most important nutrients in the human body. It is reportedly useful in the treatment of all kinds of cardiovascular diseases." After a review of the possible depletions, list the nutrients that may be depleted by the medications you are taking.

Can you identify the supplements that may interact with your medications? If not, ask a professional trained in herbal and pharmaceutical medicines, (a hard combination to find sometimes). You can also ask your pharmacist. If you find this is occurring, you must eliminate one or the other in order to maintain a safe program.

Now, identify any toxic ingredients that may be in the supplements you have been purchasing. Look specifically to avoid those dyes identified as FD&C synthetic dye numbers. Also, avoid aspartame, sugar, sucralose, talc and mineral oil. These are described on the back of the product label or on the original box, often under 'other ingredients'.

Decide within what level of cost you feel most comfortable. Understand, you will get what you pay for, but no doubt cost is a factor these days. If you can, buy the best quality you can when it comes to putting something in your body designed to benefit your health. If you go to the effort to supplement, you will want it to mean something for the good.

Begin your supplement program by looking at your lists you have just created. You should begin to see a clear picture of what you need if you have acquired the information. Start your supplementation with a good quality vitamin and mineral supplement, preferably from a capsule or powder instead of a tablet for easier absorption. Then add in the items you have identified through the lists you have made.

For heart health, you will want to make sure to have about 100 mg of CoQ10. For cancer prevention 200 – 400 mcg of selenium is essential. To keep your immune system strong, at least

500 mg of vitamin C and at least 15 mg of zinc a day is important. For good bone health you need, between food and supplemental resources, at least 1,000 mg a day of calcium depending on your age, and your sex (men need less than women).

You do not get into a car and begin to drive without first setting your destination goals; you do not plan your financial future without knowing what your end result should be; nor should you forge ahead accumulating bottles upon bottles of products you have just read about in a magazine, heard about on TV, or sold by a commissioned sales person.

Plan your work and work your plan and the rewards will be yours for life.

* * *

ARE ONE-A-DAYS ENOUGH?

The invention of the one-a-day vitamins was novel and innovative. Somewhere during a marketing meeting someone cried "Eureka," and got a hefty raise for this idea. However, nowhere has anyone said that this is all you need to be optimally healthy.

The ad that says, "Now, more complete that ever," makes me wonder, "Isn't complete already complete?" One would be led to believe that the answer is probably, no. A to Z means just that, and only that. What is misleading in many ways is the hidden message that what is in a one-a-day vitamin, taken once a day, is all we need to prevent chronic illness and help us live a long and healthy life. Unfortunately, the RDA levels are too low to overcome most medical challenges. We have come too far with orthomolecular medicine (using vitamins for therapeutic purposes) to still believe that just 60 milligrams of Vitamin C a day will keep us as well as we can possibly be.

The Recommended Dietary Allowance (RDA) was established decades ago when the focus of medicine was on illness, not on maintenance of health and vitality, and when research on nutrients was almost nonexistent. Today, we know that vitamins and minerals do more than protect us from disease. They play a key role in disease prevention and correction, given at the correct dosages, usually much higher than the RDA.

In those days, the RDA numbers were considered to be the amount of essential nutrients needed for "practically all healthy persons." These were average people who have average weight, average stress levels, average heredity patterns, and average digestive function. Who are those who *don't* meet these criteria these days? Obviously, many of us. Times have changed since the establishment of the RDA (one-a-day levels) and now those amounts are not enough to satisfy the health needs of people living in today's society.

Certainly if your doctors recommend a vitamin, follow their instructions, always checking the ingredients on the original package for any toxic dyes listed that are often found in inexpensive, over-the-counter brands (those ingredients with FD@C dye numbers such as 4, 5, 6, 40, and others). The color of the pill will be a clue to the amount of toxic dyes found in them.

It is best to couple your multi-vitamin supplement with good nutrition, as nutritionally oriented doctors suggest. But before you submit to the one-a-day concept, be sure you are already eating from a well-rounded daily meal plan, complete with the 5 fruits and vegetables recommended (a habit only 9% of Americans can actually lay claim to), making your one vitamin the *extra* protection your already optimal diet gives you, not the *only* protection.

No optimal diet? Welcome to reality. Besides those with hamburger and French fry tastes, here is a list of others who live in the real world, and need extra nutrient help: those of high or low body weight, have chronic illness, have heavy physical or emotional stress, are taking medications, have digestive problems, have wounds, burns, or injuries, are pregnant, are over age 50, and drug and alcohol abusers, just to name a few.

Each of us has our own "biochemical individuality." Environmental and lifestyle stressors and other factors can increase the need for essential nutrients beyond that which may be supplied by the SAD (Standard American Diet). Naturopathic doctors feel that Americans are slowly becoming more and more deficient of vital nutrients, developing us into a society burdened by fatigue, weight gain, and chronic illness. We work towards helping people to reestablish their bodies own ability to heal itself by suggesting the nutritional building blocks it needs to be healthy.

Choosing the right multi-vitamin, in accordance with your diet and lifestyle, is important to not only being well, but staying well. If you choose to be "A to Z complete," though, make sure your *first* choice is to be completely "H" . . . for healthy.

* * *

CALCIUM: DOUBLED EDGED SWORD

When is the calcium in an antacid pill not a complete bone-building formula? All of the time.

Despite published research that describes the full spectrum of nutrients needed for total bone health (mainly minerals), many people still rely on a one-stop supplement to take care of both bone and belly.

No doubt buying calcium supplements is as confusing as buying pantyhose. They come in a variety of packages, describe varying sizes (dosages), and all brands claim to fit your needs, often times requiring the head-scratching, time-consuming, stand-and-study process at the retail store shelves.

Some doctors are still recommending calcium supplements that also serve as antacids, to women who need calcium after menopause for maintain bone strength. It is a quick and easy solution to two problems at once, they feel. However, let's take a closer look by reading the back label of a popular antacid/calcium resource.

Now, understand I am not picking on one brand or another, only calcium carbonate supplements, and those brands used as both an antacid and a calcium bone-building supplement, as one particular 'get two-in-one' product label describes.

This particular brand offers warnings and drug interaction precautions on the "antacid" side. We are not to take the "maximum dosage" of this product for more than two weeks, it says, except under the advice and supervision of a physician. In addition, we need to know that antacids may interact with certain prescription drugs. "If you are presently taking prescription drug," the label reads, "do not take the product without checking with your physician or healthcare professional." Good to know.

On the "calcium supplement" side of this label, we are directed to use this product as a source of "extra calcium," not necessarily as our complete daily calcium requirement. The label continues to say in bold print, "A balanced diet with enough calcium and regular exercise throughout life will help you to build and maintain healthy bones and may reduce your risk of developing osteoporosis." And since this company provides grant money to the National Osteoporosis Foundation (also on the label), they ought to know.

And while we are talking labels, let us read further to note that this particular label lists sugar (sucrose) as its main ingredient, as well as talc, and mineral oil, plus four dyes that have been

120

studied and shown to be toxic to some people. It is no wonder the label also says, "Keep out of the reach of children."

Why do I not like the action of an antacid combined with the action of a bone-building calcium supplement? Simple. It is true that calcium carbonate neutralizes acid in the stomach thereby being an effective antacid. Unfortunately, we need our stomach acid to dissolve and absorb calcium and other minerals for our health. Consequently, by over-neutralizing our stomach acid with an antacid, we might not absorb the very calcium we thought we were taking if for, for bone health. Yes, calcium carbonate is the cheapest form of calcium, since it literally is just chalk, and it does actually contain more calcium than other forms. But current research is showing other calcium "forms" may be much better dissolved and absorbed, the key factor for reaching the important target locations, the bones.

There seems to be no definitive research on which form is best for all people, but I tend to line up with those studies showing significant bone thickness increases with people having taken a complete bone-mineral formula, as compared to those who just take the one mineral, calcium, by itself.

A fairly unknown type of calcium, microcrystalline hydroxyapatite concentrate (MCHC), is a well-absorbed calcium source and contains mineral other than calcium that are involved in bone formation: phosphorus, fluoride, magnesium, iron, zinc, copper, manganese, and others. MCHC is actual bone, itself, so it contains all the vital components important to a healthy skeleton. All MCHC products are not created equally, however, so check with a medical doctor trained in natural medicine for their product recommendation.

Not only is calcium carbonate not the best source as a bone-nourishing supplement, it is not a complete bone food. It may be malabsorbed by those with compromised intestinal health, and its antacid effect may interfere with good digestion. By shutting down our stomach acid, we easier entertain growth of harmful bacteria and yeast that normally will not flourish in the acidic stomach environment with which nature has provided us for this very bacterial-killing purpose.

Bacteria and yeast overgrowth leads to GI gas, bloating, diarrhea, and abdominal pain. Eliminating stomach acid also prevents some foods from being digested, creating food putrification in the intestines, and prevents some vitamins (which need acid to "break" the molecule) and minerals from being absorbed, leading to fatigue from lack of B vitamin absorption and other physical symptoms from mineral deficiencies.

The take home message here is if you want to reduce your stomach acid, take a look at the foods you are eating that may be creating the problem in the first place and the stressful conditions under which you are eating them, and change those first. (Chewing gum also stimulates stomach acids, sometimes causing "GERD" symptoms, as the chewing mouth alerts the stomach for the food it thinks is coming, but never does.)

Before you decide to neutralize your stomach acid while trying to dissolve your calcium source, try this experiment. Put one of your calcium antacids in a small bowl of water (no acid), and another one in a small bowl of vinegar (very acid). See which dissolves and which sits there doing nothing. Granted that since your stomach acid is acidic, you get good break down and dissolving. But, as it becomes less acidic (water)…well, you will see.

If you insist on taking calcium carbonate for bone-building calcium, take it with meals when your stomach acid is high during digestion. However, if taking the calcium as an antacid, you should not be taking it during meals to shut the acid down, since you need your stomach acid for good digestion and vital nutrient absorption. Confusing, I know. 'Best rule-of-thumb is to not take an antacid at all.

My advice for your best health is to eliminate the antacids whenever possible. Focus on other ways to reduce elevated stomach acid, by addressing what is really knawing at you, and pick a calcium form that you can take any time of day and still get good absorption (calcium citrate or MCHC).

Throw out your bone-and-belly pills, and both bone and belly will thank you.

* * *

DRUG THERAPY: WHAT'S MISSING FROM THIS PICTURE?

There's an emerging body of scientific data that is telling us that side effects often experienced from pharmaceuticals may not only be from their toxic effects on the body, but perhaps a result of the nutrient deficiencies they are causing.

So far, few doctors are considering nutrient-depletions as causes for our fatigue. We lay blame on lack of sleep or stress, but maybe it is the missing B vitamins that have been depleted from a medication commonly being taken. Or it could be a lacking mineral, essential for making the biochemical energy 'sparkplug' that is causing a fatigue-related health problem.

Drug-induced nutrient depletion is a concept rarely taken into account in today's conventional allopathic healthcare. Most medical doctors are not aware of this problem, since their drug reps either don't know, or are unwilling to tell them about it. And although pharmacists would be a good resource for these answers, they may be hesitant to offer the information for similar reasons. There are, however, scientific studies that support that this is becoming a problem. It is shocking to me that the drug aimed at correcting a medical problem, is depleting the very nutrient that organ system needs to be healthy.

Nutrient depletions cause real health problems. A subject not studied expensively in conventional medical school, medical nutrition (biochemistry) is the foundation of health and wellness. If not considered as part of an overall health program, it will leave one incomplete and without the full resources to return to their optimal health. It is bad enough that our soils often do not supply us with the vital minerals we need for health. But now we have to factor in the depletions caused by our "health program" as provided by medications.

Does this sound far-fetched? Yes, and scary, too. Does anyone wonder why heart disease and cancer is so out-of-control? Do you wonder why heart disease is more rampant with women than with men?

Perhaps it is the heart-healthy nutrients, including folic acid, being depleted by the estrogens from first the oral birth control pills, then later the hormone replacement. Add to that the extra deficiencies of folic acid caused by pain medications such as Aleve, Advil, Motrin, and Celebrex and we begin seeing increased rates of anemia and other cardiovascular diseases.

Unless nutrient deficiencies are being considered as the cause, most drug companies shake their head and say, "We don't know why this is happening." Their studies do not assess nutrient deficiencies, consequently, they can report "improvements," from taking the drug, while in the meantime, the body's DNA could be suffering from damage, or the cellular structures could be changing, neither of which are checked with common lab work or considered in their company-sponsored study.

In order to appreciate this huge health problem, a health provider must understand the role nutrients have on the body and the consequences of their depleted states. In some areas of the country where naturopathic medicine is common, clinical discussions on drug-induced depletions are common. However, in areas where there is a lack of natural medicine knowledge, it goes unknown and is never considered as an easy and inexpensive solution to health repair.

Some common symptoms due to nutrient depletions include depression, fatigue, muscle and joint pain, dry skin, heart palpitations, dizziness, insomnia, and frequent illness. Conditions and diseases related to nutrient deficiencies include heart attacks and disease, osteoporosis, fibromyalgia, cancer, anemia, macular degeneration, and high blood pressure.

Hopefully, word will begin to spread that there exists a large and credible body of scientific data relating to drug-induced nutrient deficiencies. Theoretically, it should begin with the drug producers themselves. Surprisingly, a leading cholesterol drug manufacturer not only knows of the nutrient depletion caused by its drug, it holds a patent on a combination product that actually puts it back in. Unfortunately, it has never been introduced or offered to the public.

And although many medical experts are aware of this nutrient-depleting situation and have repeatedly informed the FDA of the harmful health effects the drug is having on people's health due to this nutrient depletion, the FDA has done nothing to address it, nor insist that the drug company make it available in its product.

Now that we can begin to understand, "What is missing from this picture," we should begin to ask, "What is *wrong* with this picture?"

* * *

HOLIDAY & TRAVEL

FOR THE NATURAL-AT-HEART TRAVEL KIT

Whether it is off to the beach, off to Florida, or heading to Europe it is best to be prepared for times when calling the doctor is not as easy as it often is at home.

I know from experience that a call to the local 'medicine man' in an unfamiliar town may present you with a situation where the two of you do not speak the same language, either literally or figuratively. Best to bring your medical resources with you, and you know I mean those of the natural kind.

Number one on my list of 'always take with me' is zinc. At the first sign of a "bug," 15 – 25 mg of this mineral three times a day with food will help prevent you from coming down with something. If you can find a formula that adds goldenseal and vitamin C with citrus bioflavonoids, all the better.

A soothing salve is great for overexposure to the sun, chapped lips, or just keeping skin smooth from abrasions. A small 1-ounce tub formulated with creamy vitamin E, lavender oil, and calendula will feel great and comes in handy for many purposes. A little witch hazel over an insect sting, cut, or poison ivy blister before you dab on the salve will offer even more pain relief. For those a bit more adventurous, a tiny bit of ammonia over an unrelenting itch will give you great relief.

For stomach upsets, there are many items to have on hand to get you past the acute stages. For diarrhea, a formula with bismuth (the active ingredient in Pepto-Bismol®) is great, coupled with a natural anti-microbial called berberine. In addition, strange as it is, a substance called bentonite (yes, clay) or activated charcoal can help remove toxins that may be the aggravating problem to begin with.

For constipation herbs like senna, cascara sagrada, or triphala work well. A good dose of magnesium (400 milligrams) at night will also relax the smooth muscles in your bowel to help you move your bowels.

The best anti-microbial prevention, though, is to keep your hands washed. Always have a tube of anti-microbial cleansing gel in the car, or your purse, and use it frequently, as getting to a clean restroom is not always a choice. Many people like the anti-microbial protection that grapefruit seed extract (GSE) offers. This fluid can be used topically and internally to help kill bacteria, but always read the labels and make sure to dilute before using, as it is quite strong.

If you are going on a long jaunt and want to reduce the number of supplements you are going to take, make your priority list based on your existing medical conditions. (Always keep all of your doctor-prescribed medicines on you, where you can get to them should your bags get lost.) During both short and long trips, I advise maintaining good supplementation of the B vitamins for sustained energy, vitamin E for continual good blood flow through veins and brain, and vitamin C to help ward off infections of others you may come in contact with too closely.

A good herbal relaxant like valerian root or a few milligrams of melatonin is good to have available at night so that proper rest can be assured. (It is always good to check with your doctor before embarking on these herbals therapies.) And if you do not know how much to take, or whether or not they will interact with your current medicines, DO NOT take them.

Above all, bring your kava kava, and make sure you can get to it easily. You will be glad you had your natural anti-anxiety herb on you when they tell you your flight has been cancelled, that you will miss your connection, and you realize that you forgot to bring your favorite book. Relax, breathe, and remember how good it is sometimes just stay at home.

* * *

GIVE THE GIFT OF HEALTH

Still scratching your head about what to give this year for Christmas? Whether as stocking stuffers, or for placement under the tree, give some serious thought to a gift for those you love, geared toward health improvement.

A good multiple vitamin and mineral formula from a reputable resource can be just what the doctor ordered. Choose one in capsule form (dissolves well in your stomach), and one that does not have too much iron in it. Also, check the ingredients and avoid any that indicate yellow, blue, or red dyes or sugars as these can deplete health, not improve it.

Postmenopausal women will be benefited with the addition of hormone balancing herbs in the formula, such as black cohosh, vitex agnes, dong quai, or sage. Men over age 50 will appreciate finding a prostate-protecting formula with saw palmetto included.

Most everyone could use a good B-complex vitamin formula. Always take B vitamins in "complex" form, since these vitamins are best absorbed into the body when taken together. One-a-day of a high-quality formula should help decrease fatigue, depression, insomnia, and anemia among many other health conditions. Always choose B vitamins and folic acid in their 'active forms' since a large percent of the population cannot metabolize in their bodies the 'cheaper' forms of vitamins. They need to be in their methylated forms to assure absorption due to a DNA mutation commonly seen in many people. (If you are unfamiliar with the activated forms of B vitamins and folic acid, it will be worth your while to do the research to learn.)

Books are good this year for giving. There are many books on herbal medicine that are colorful and entertaining, not to mention helpful in supplying important basic information in staving off illness. One that I especially like is *Prescription for Nutritional Healing* by Balch and Balch. It offers a naturopathic list of therapies on a multitude of conditions, is easy to read, and extensive in its offering of information.

Creams and lotions are great to give to someone who may return the gift of massage to you. Look for those with vitamin E or other natural oils for the best healing properties. Avoid those with mineral oil or petroleum. Even though these ingredients usually make the product less expensive, they tend to clog the skin more than they nourish it. Always warm the cream in your own hands first before you apply it to another person. A cold blob of cream falling on a bare back can be less than relaxing, even if it was well-intended by the giver.

Exercise CDs are available. There are many good ones that require only a small space in our home for their use. Some focus on dancing, a great anti-depression aid, some on walking, good for lowering cholesterol, and others focus on yoga stretching positions, demonstrating how spinal flexibility supports better health.

As sugar plums dance through our heads, and chocolate Santas can be heard saying "and to all a good night," don't forget what you have learned about eating sweets this year.

When you care to give the very best, make it a gift of health. Meeting our healthy New Year's resolutions will just be that much easier to achieve.

* * *

Nature does not hurry, yet everything is accomplished

LAO TZU

CREATING HEART-HEALTHY RECIPES FOR THE HOLIDAYS

All too often, we forget to protect the very life-preserving functions that keep us alive; on top of the list is our heart. We get busy, grabbing a fast food here and a processed food there, not thinking what we are doing to our health and longevity. Even though we may know what the right choice is, sometimes it seems as though our brains, and our decision-making abilities, are not connected to the rest of our bodies. Over time, this habitual 'loss of consciousness' could make us sick, or worse, cut short our life.

Conventional medical training does not often stress the connection between the digestive and cardiovascular systems. Each seems to be separate systems with their own pathologies, diagnoses, and medications. However, as the world of healthcare evolves into integrative medicine, we begin to acknowledge more and more that what we eat becomes an important part of our biochemistry.

Knowing that even a little education on heart health can turn into extra years with our friends and family, here is some information on food choices that can provide that heart health support most of us need.

Let us begin to apply this knowledge through the selection of fats and oils. Experts are now saying that the key to finding a truly healthy diet seems to be centered not so much on its total amount of fat, but more on the type of fat being ingested. By monitoring our cholesterol levels and dietary cholesterol-rich food sources, without consideration for the health of our coronary arteries, we may be missing important information. Cholesterol is not all bad; it is essential to the manufacturing of other important hormones in the body including testosterone and estrogen.

Before dietary fats and oils get to the liver after eating a meal, they travel from the lining of the small intestine of the digestive system, absorbed into the lymphatic system that flows into the veins that feed blood directly into the heart. Can we then assume that saturated fats, trans-fatty acids, and old rancid oils might end up in the heart and its associated arterial system? Yes.

To avoid this chance of forming arterial plaque deposits (atherosclerosis), choose olive oil when preparing recipes and food sources rich in omega-3 fatty acid oils, such as fish, avoiding excessive amounts of high-saturated foods like the animal foods of bacon, butter, lard, and hamburger meat. Although, according to Dr. Andrew Weil and many others, it is better to eat butter than margarine.

If we were to continue to design a heart healthy holiday, we would want to include foods rich in flavonoids. Flavonoids and bioflavonoids are special plant nutrients (phytochemicals) found abundantly in the plant kingdom. One may identify a flavonoid by the terms commonly used such as hesperidin, quercitin, rutin, catechin, pine bark extract, and OPCs (grape seed extract). These have been used in Europe for centuries as natural medicinal agents for improving circulation and strengthening the membranes of blood vessels and capillaries.

Grape flavonoids act as natural blood thinners, helpful in preventing blood clots. Grapefruit and orange juice are also rich in flavonoids, but comparison studies have shown that purple grape juice, the grape seed and skin extract, appears to be better for the heart by reducing blood platelet (the clotting cell) 'stickiness.' Other flavonoid-strong foods are blueberries, bilberries, and cranberries.

Nuts and seeds can be both hearty and healthy. Ground flax seeds can easily be added to a holiday recipe. Some studies have shown omega-3 flax seed and oil to have a cholesterol-managing effect, increasing the healthy HDLs, and having a lowering effect for high blood pressure, as well. Some experts say that supplementing selenium with the omega-3 oils will improve its action.

Add raw almonds to your favorite holiday taste treat, as well. Clinical studies support eating a handful of almonds a day, saying that this will decrease the bad cholesterol, the LDLs. Nuts contain plant sterols, such as 'beta sitosterol,' that account for their cholesterol lowering behavior.

Don't forget to add the celery to a stuffing recipe or casserole. Celery has been used therapeutically by Asian cultures for centuries to lower blood pressure and often is responsible for lower cholesterol as well.

Think of this bountiful nutrient-rich cornucopia when planning your holiday health-providing recipes, and know that your heart (and your family) will be thanking you.

* * *

HEALING

FIBROMYALGIA: FACT OR FICTION?

One of the most complex and difficult to treat conditions, fibromyalgia and its causes, still remain a mystery. A condition characterized by chronic body pain, depression, irritable bowel syndrome, headaches, sleep disturbances, just to name a few, fibromyalgia syndrome is not understood even by most doctors. Often dismissed as being only "in the head" of the patients, those suffering from this debilitating condition want and need more help than that which is commonly offered.

Complicated as it is, it takes more than a typical 10-minute office visit to accurately diagnose and treat fibromyalgia. If the physical exam is performed properly, nine pairs of tender point on the body will be present, plus a long list of other ailments. Obtaining a history of antibiotic use is important, saliva testing to determine levels of hormones is helpful, and complete lab work can also be diagnostic.

Taking a diet history is also essential given the correlations suggesting that fibromyalgia is possibly associated with candida (yeast) overgrowth, irritable bowel syndrome, and malabsorption. And given the close proximity of the source of the pain to the neck and the common symptom of chronic headaches, a serious consideration should be given to chiropractic techniques that could, in fact, be corrective.

It is no wonder that drug-based conventional medicine has not found the source of the problem. Given its multi-dimensional properties, it is a "whole body" condition, and its correction may lie in assisting the body to heal itself, removing the obstacles to health, not just medicating it with drugs, as is commonly done. True, there are exceptionally effective drugs that can lighten a depression, help one to sleep, and remove the pain. However, wouldn't the ultimate and best solution be to avoid a lifetime of dependency on those drugs? It is, of course, everyone's personal choice.

Those doctors who do understand the tragic dilemma those with fibromyalgia face and who are sympathetic and active in helping to find its resolve, know that it requires more than drugs to get a handle on the solution if they want to see improvement in their patients. They know that by working closely with their patients, they often times can slowly unravel the cause or causes that have created, perhaps over long term, these symptoms in the first place. These doctors have knowledge of toxic elements, foods, and know that even an excess of some commonly supplemented minerals can often cause pain.

Information on nutrients that support muscle health, how hormones can be brought back to normal ranges to reduce depression, and ways to help eliminate fatigue are all being utilized in medicine by a few doctors for curative results.

The cause of fibromyalgia is multifaceted, and yes, complicated. It seems to be the culmination and manifestation of hormone and nutrient deficiencies, the result of injury or stress, spinal imbalances, and of toxicity in the body. The road to recovery is a process of resolving one situation at a time. With time, and patience, it can be done.

* * *

Healing is a matter of time,
but it is sometimes also
a matter of opportunity.
HIPPOCRATES

LIGHT A CANDLE FOR YOURSELF

In response to recent events, we are all looking for a way to help, desperate for a grasp on reality, searching for a way to control our destiny and affect a positive result for our futures. An invisible force has swept down on us, like a hidden hive of killer bees, attacking us at our most vulnerable spot, shaking our faith and trust in knowing that we can relax because all is well.

We are now on alert to the hidden hives that still may be haunting our very neighborhoods, having to be constantly aware to what may be just around the corner, always watching for a sign that may put us on the run.

This is no way to live, and certainly this hyper-vigilance is harmful to our health. There is much talk and advice about going about our lives, remaining unaffected by those whose intent is to place fear in our hearts and rob us of our well-being. Yet, there is a yearning to do something to help, to contribute to those who are suffering, to aid in the recovery. Many are frustrated in their attempts to express their helpful energies, not knowing what to do; some rebel through anger; others retreat into silence. Since often we are left with few options, we light a candle and say a prayer for those who have been directly and indirectly affected in an attempt to participate and support those who are hurting.

I suggest we light a candle for ourselves. Not only does health begin at home, but when we are strong, we can be strong for others. If we are not conscious of our physical well-being at this time, we could see a widespread health decline in the coming weeks and months. Our immune systems will take a tumble, our bodies will become depleted of important nutrients. If we do not continue to eat and rest, fatigue could set in from stress and sleepless nights, and the enemy will have gained some points from our demise. It is a subtle strike, and one that few are thinking of, but one that we cannot allow. If we do not address it now, our dampened spirits could slowly drain us of our vitality, creating physical weakening in a time we need to be strong.

Make your personal health plan and commit to it now. This is how you can contribute, this is how you can regain control, and affect a positive result for our future. Here are a few essentials that we all need to do to keep ourselves from illness as a result of the intense stress and sadness we have had to endure:

Spend some quiet time reflecting on what health conditions you have been ignoring; have your notebook in hand. Make a list of the aches, pains, and concerns that are aggravating or worrisome. Then list under each of these symptoms actions that you are taking to resolve or relieve each problem. Look at your eating habits and make an effort to make the right food choices to maintain your strength and energy.

Check in with your doctor, especially if you have not done so for a while. Get a complete blood work-up and make a plan that will realign abnormal values. Keep your blood pressure normal. Nourish and lift your spirits by doing random acts of kindness.

Breathe slowly and deeply. Start a regular exercise program. Keep your immune system strong, especially as cold and flu season draws near. Practice preventive medicine, as an ounce of prevention is worth a pound of cure.

As a naturopathic physician this last idea, of course, is my favorite suggestion. If we are not cognizant of the passing of time, and our existence through it, we will find the clock has ticked away faster than we have realized. Now is the time to secure and protect our long-term health with serious and methodical attention to it, working actively towards our goals. Plan your work and work your plan. This not only means taking the medications we need that could save our life, but also supporting our health with the basis of health itself, the healing power of nature. And whatever that means for each individual, now is the time to embrace it.

I have put aside discussing my usual health concerns such as dust mites, dog bites, and imbalanced electrolytes to address this very serious subject. A call to arms is at hand, and as we kiss our loved ones good-bye, and light a candle for their safe return, let us then turn to light our own candle, remembering that in this calm before the storm, we have a job at home to do - that of keeping ourselves strong and healthy and safe from illness. United - and healthy - we stand.

We owe it to ourselves, our families, and as a tribute to and in honor of those who are now so much in our thoughts and prayers.

* * *

There are two ways of spreading light:
To be the candle,
Or the mirror that reflects it.

LET PEACE BEGIN WITH ME

There's a beautiful song that says, "Let peace begin with me." It is an especially important message for these times, as it requires each of us to first find the peace within us, and demonstrates its value to others through peaceful example.

With the events of September 11 not worn off yet, we find ourselves confronted with even more stress, that of "preparing for Christmas." Have we gone too crazy preparing for an event that should flow naturally, gracefully, and lovingly?

The first Christmas was simple, joyous, and peaceful. No loud crowds, no road rage, and no list of have-to-dos to rush to complete. The "decorations" were of natural wood and hay, illuminated with natural lighting and scented with barn animals in the fresh evening air. Gifts were hand delivered with love, not sent packed in plastic peanuts. The shepherds did not push, yell, and shove to the front of the line to meet a postal deadline, but were no doubt calmly excited, respectful of the occasion.

Can we imagine the peace and tranquility that was present that first Christmas night? Can we picture it and hold that image firmly in our thoughts? What good does it do to become impatient standing in line, lose our cool, and upset with those who are trying to help us? To what peaceful or joyous purpose does that serve?

To help manage these potential surges of irritation, here are some helpful ideas:

Avoid the sugary treats. Eating them creates hyper-activity, otherwise known as "bouncing off the walls," and will only add to your risk of illness. Sugar depletes our immune system, and robs us of the important vitamins our body needs to stay well. Stress will do the same. Put the two together and you set yourself up for frequent attacks of colds and flu, not to mention more fatigue.

Balance work with play. Dr. Sigmund Freud said the average person needs eight hours of work and two hours of fun every day in order to maintain good mental health.

Focus on the positive, not the negative; focus on the solution, not the problem. Focusing on the positive will magnify and multiply it. It has been said that the greatest weapon against stress is the ability to choose one thought over another.

Get assistance with difficult matters. A fresh pair of eyes, an objective second opinion, a sympathetic ear, or a shoulder to cry on may be just what the doctor ordered to help you get through the rest of the holidays.

Perhaps becoming stress-free this time of year is easier said than done. When there are Christmas morning expectations from eager children, social events happening, and Christmas decorations awaiting their seasonal placements throughout the house, it can indeed be fun to participate.

What we must avoid, however, is for our own physical, mental, and emotional well-being turning from fun into frenzy. We can bet the Wise Men did not act from stress and frenzy as they arrived at their Christmas scene; they would have destroyed the magic of the moment.

Therefore, it should be with us these days, as well. Slow down. Greet your neighbors and family, do not run them down. Wish them a happy holiday; do not ruin their holiday with your stress. Be considerate. Be patient. Keep it simple. Get your rest. Laugh. You will enjoy smiling more than you will yell. Relax and enjoy these days. They were meant for celebration and peace, not designed to be a Hollywood production.

Remember the words, "Let there be peace on Earth and let it begin with me. Let there be peace on Earth, the kind that was meant to be. With God as our Father, brothers all are we. Let us walk with each other, in perfect harmony. Let peace begin with me."

* * *

If we open a quarrel between the past and the present,
We shall find that we have lost the future.

WINSTON CHURCHILL

TIME TO TURN THE TURTLE AROUND

Have you been slow to make health changes this year? Have you gradually been crawling down the wrong road, not seeing the forest for the trees, getting deeper and deeper, lost in the darkness of disease?

If so, it is time to turn the turtle around. That which has crept slowly into ill health, can slowly creep back. What is important, however, is to be pointed in the right direction, turtle-speed or not.

It is easy to give up and feel that the return path to good health is long and hard. We are programmed to look for quick change and immediate results. However, when we look at the "speed of nature," we note slow, not fast, change. It is this very pace, which we should match as our pace, expecting no less and no more.

With the holidays winding down, here are some health tips we need to be focusing on now, while preparing for a commitment to better health as part of our New Year's resolutions.

Start by forgiving yourself for all the over-indulgences of which you are guilty these last few weeks, knowing that life is to be enjoyed, but that good health comes from good food choices. Begin to throw out, yes THROW OUT, foods that you love, but do not love you. These are the candies that are getting old, the turkey that may be harboring bacteria, and the eggnog, alcohol, and pop that is not getting any more sugar-free by being in your house. Throw away old holiday cookies, fruitcake, and fudge that are now part of the past, turning the turtle around now to better days. Do not consider giving them to "the kids." They are just as bad, if not worse, for them.

Start replacing your food supply with multi-grain breads, chicken, beans, hearty cereals, and low-fat milk. Instead of continuing to drink the whole milk upon which you have been raised, try a low fat or skim milk, or even be adventurous and try the soymilk or almond milk.

Begin adding raisins, oats, ground flax and milk thistle seed, wheat germ, and high protein raw almonds and walnuts to existing boxed cereals to fortify them with extra vitamins, minerals, and fiber. Mix up all ingredients and keep in an airtight plastic box for scooping out any time of day for a meal or snack.

Get back on your supplement program. With all the rushing around from holiday agendas, it is sometimes hard to remember that supplements, especially if specifically designed for your health by a health care practitioner, are a must for your optimal health. Refill those that are gone, and recommit to your original supplement program. It may also be time to review and make changes to a plan that is over a year old, as times change and people change. Check expiration dates; throw out any that are expired. Same with medications.

Begin to decrease your sugar intake. Start by limiting it during five straight days a week, allowing little more leniencies over the weekend. This includes alcohol, vending machine candy, soft drinks, sweet rolls, and jelly on your toast. Not to be excluded is the sugar you add to the coffee though the day, and the sugar in the sweet tea you drink. It all adds up; it is hard on insulin control, and leads to an increase in sugar-cravings. Start now to eliminate the sugar, breaking the habit of eating it, and eventually your craving for it will be gone. Once you begin eliminating it from your body, you will want it less. Sugar is a poison and we can become addicted to its taste and effects on the body. Start to detox now.

Start reading package labels. Make this another healthy habit. Avoid products that contain Yellow Dye #5 or #6, or any other color additive. Strangely enough, many over-the-counter supplements contain toxic dyes. Many people are allergic to them and some artificial dyes have actually found to be cancer-causing over time. Also, avoid hydrogenated, or partially hydrogenated, oils. These are toxic, chemically-changed oil molecules that add to their life on the shelf, but not to our life on this earth. You will find this mostly in packaged foods.

Lift your spirits and keep them there. Although easy to say, it often requires practice by doing it over time in order to maintain a strong positive attitude. Do not give in to seasonal depression because "you can." Break the cycle now. Focus on the positive, multiplying its energy. Do not give power to negativity, as it does not belong to a healthy mind, body, or spirit. Couple that with forgiveness and random acts of kindness and there will be no room for depression.

Begin to plant the thought of what long-term health goals you would like to accomplish this year. If you have been hiding under a shell, hoping no one will notice your slow demise into ill health and insist that you make a change, if you have been crawling in the wrong direction and you know it, time to turn the turtle around.

* * *

Be not afraid of growing slowly;
Be afraid of standing still.

CHINESE PROVERB

RETURN TO GOOD HEALTH BY GIVING TO YOURSELF

If you are like most people through the holidays, your joy has come from giving generously to others. You may have sacrificed your time, your money, and perhaps even your energy so that those you love and care about could experience some holiday fun, good treats to eat, and a variety of blessings of abundance. And certainly, it is from giving that we also receive. Perhaps, though, you have also sacrificed your health.

Sacrificing "some" for others is a virtue, but sacrificing "all" is a mistake. Are you the provider to family or friends all year long, as well? Stop and ask yourself how much you save back to give yourself. What do you give yourself to sustain your health that keeps you strong and free of chronic illness while you are so graciously giving to others? If the answer is "nothing", perhaps your dispersement of time and money and list of priorities may need a second look because giving everything away, retaining nothing for your own mental, physical, or financial well-being may not be the best of practices.

Decide what your long term (or short term) goals are. Give some thought and jot some notes on how you plan to reach those goals. Now, make a list of your most pressing priorities, or sources of stress, listing the benefits that acting upon them will bring. By postponing action on those stress-producing irritants, the "residue" related to their constant presence will eventually manifest in ill health.

Write down the ways that giving to yourself, addressing mind-consuming issues, and avoiding what is harmful or unsupportive of your goals will benefit your total health and longevity.

Next, decide what is depleting your health the most this very day. This could include emotional health, financial health, or physical health. Are we afraid to act, or just afraid to look at the problem? It has been said that when we face the Dragon, the Dragon will go away. Think about what issues you have not dealt with, that if addressed and acted upon would make you feel better instantly. Has there been a family confrontation that with a simple, "I'm sorry," could mend a wound? Is your schedule too busy that you find yourself giving up too much of your energy and not saving enough for your own daily repair or healing? If so, make some changes now.

Many of you have heard me say that the healthiest word in the dictionary is, "No." Declining a few requests of others may not make much of an actual difference to them, but might make a huge difference in the long run to your overall well-being. Try it. It is not as hard to say "no" as one would think. Giving away too much of ourselves does not leave us with much of a slice from the pie chart of our own lives. Is that what you are choosing to do, or just what you are doing "automatically"? Stop and think and let your actions and choices become "conscious" again.

Make a list of your food choices during the last month; yes, last month. It may be these foods that if not changed now may lead to your ill health. We have had enough candy, enough alcohol, enough fruitcake, and enough cookies to last us until next holiday season. Sugar depletes our immune system and robs us of the energy-producing benefits of B vitamins. Sugar also feeds bacteria, yeast, and cancer cells.

Stop the sugar now. Replace these disease-producing foods with strong emphasis for a few weeks on raw, steamed, or baked vegetables (except corn), and some hearty soups of beans and peas, which include extra amounts of garlic, onions, and olive oil. Throw your left over goodies away and begin to be health conscious again. This includes the kids' old holiday candy, too. There is no time better than the present to begin to teach them proper food choices and lifestyle habits.

It is time now to give back on track. In a previous article, I wrote about how if we had not addressed a developing chronic condition by the end of the year, it was "time to turn the turtle around," and begin to head back to the Road to Good Health. Same song, second verse for some of us this year. Although permanent change is a slow and constant process, once back on track, things can only get better.

Giving to oneself is an act of self-love and is especially hard for those who love easily and give so generously, as it requires saving some love back for themselves. Just remember that although what you give comes back ten-fold, sometimes it is not what you give away, but what you keep for yourself that may bring you your best health rewards.

* * *

AFTERWORD

MESSAGES OF "THANKS" - TAKE SOME AND PASS IT ON

Although unconditional love helps to open doors to Eternal Life, and forgiveness is the cornerstone to health and happiness, saying thanks to those who have helped us is the foundation that secures our good relationships with friends and family in the present.

As we begin our holiday hustle and bustle, let us take a Claus-pause to think of those who have given of themselves to make our lives easier. I believe we create ill fate, or bad "karma," for ourselves if we forget this important gesture. So often, we take our gifts of help for granted, expecting them to be there over and over, without our acknowledgement. This year, let us make a special effort to look around and give credit where credit is due. Saying "thanks" should be easy and helps assure continued support from those receiving the acknowledgement.

In lieu of sending hundreds of thank you cards to those I am thankful to, let me take this public opportunity to thank you all now, and encourage everyone to identify those to whom you are thankful and to pass on this same gesture.

I thank those in the Sanford medical community who have supported me and the philosophies of naturopathic medicine, and those who have helped their patients discover the power and importance of involvement in their own healthcare. Special thanks to Dr. Robert W. Patterson, MD, who believed in me and helped to bring the opportunity for optimal wellness to the people of Sanford.

Thanks to the editorial staff at the Sanford Herald who created this *'Health and Science'* page, in order that the Sanford community could be in touch with complementary and alternative medicine, through my 'Healing Power of Nature' column, as healthcare takes on new meaning throughout the country.

To Central Carolina Community College, thanks for continuing to include my classes in the course selections.

In this time of giving and saying "thanks," I especially want to recognize and acknowledge those who have worked with me personally, and those of you who are loyal readers of my column, as you work toward your goal to achieve better health. I congratulate each and every one of you for your interest and commitment to yourself. I applaud your strength and courage to look "outside the box." Thank you for your continued support. I will return your support with mine.

Thanks to my mother and my brothers - Bob Yerby and Phil Yerby - with whom I developed my personal ethics and values during the early years of my life. The memories of these experiences - of learning the meaning of good character through self-responsibility and honesty, the importance of quality nutrition from Mom's home-cooking, and the significance of being selfless by being connected to a Higher Power - will stay with me forever.

And to my North Carolina family - Terence, Martha Ray and O'Neil Shepherd - some extra big thanks and hugs for helping me feel at home in North Carolina. It has meant a lot to me to have your help, kindness, and friendship.

Often it can be difficult to thank those who we really want to recognize due to a number of complicated reasons. Sometimes time constraints, personality conflicts, or previous transgressions can cause hesitation. If that is the case, take this chance to thank them now. Get a little box of blank cards at Hallmark, write a brief note, add a smiley face or draw a heart, and sign it with a warm sentiment. Send these cards to those with whom you want to reconnect or say 'thanks'. By this gesture, you will have acknowledged their help and have expressed your appreciation, in your own private way.

This year we can celebrate the holidays and begin anew by thanking God for our blessings, and by saying thanks to the friends and family who deserve to be remembered. Do not let time go by without stopping to acknowledge the gratitude we feel for the help they have given.

Once this is accomplished, can complete forgiveness and unconditional love be far behind?

* * *

The best thing about the future,
Is that it comes one day at a time.

ABRAHAM LINCOLN

SELF-CARE RESOURCES

For Medical-Grade Product Ordering:
Dr Supplement Store   1-877-846-7122
www.DSSorders.com/OHR No-fee registration authorization CY411

Dr. Yerby's Cold and Flu Protocol - Product Suggestions:
- Thorne Research, Double Strength Zinc
- ProThera, Ester-C Bio OR Thorne Research, Vitamin C with Flavonoids
- Gaia Herbs / Professional Solutions, Black Elderberry Syrup, 5.4 fl ounces
- Wise Woman Herbals, Lomatium, 2 fl ounces

For Self-Ordering Blood Work:
www.DirectLabs.com/OHR   1-800-908-0000
(Look for the 'Monthly Specials')
Lab profile suggestions:
- CWP (Complete Wellness Profile)
- Thyroid Panel, Special (TSH, T4, and Free T3)
- Vitamin D3, 25 Hydroxy

For Restorative Formulations Products:
www.RestorativeFormulations.com   1-800-420-5801
Register on 'Create Patient Account' –Validate doctor's phone number as 919-704-6298
When talking with a customer service rep, ask for the patient-referral department when ordering.
Product Suggestions:
- Metabolic Nutrition
- Vitamin D3 10,000
- Ubiqinol 100 mg IU

Southwest College of Naturopathic Medicine and Health Sciences, Tempe, Arizona
www.SCNM.edu

American Association of Naturopathic Physicians
www.naturopathic.org

For other articles or books by Christie C. Yerby ND, search by author's name:
www.LEF.org   Life Extension Magazine / Search bar: Christie C. Yerby
www.Amazon.com/books   Search bar: Christie C. Yerby

"Ignore your health, and it will go away."

www.ingramcontent.com/pod-product-compliance
Lightning Source LLC
Chambersburg PA
CBHW081127170526
45165CB00008B/2576